THE RADIOLOGY
OF ACUTE CERVICAL
SPINE TRAUMA

THE RADIOLOGY OF ACUTE CERVICAL SPINE TRAUMA

John H. Harris, Jr., M.D., D.Sc.

Chairman, Department of Radiology
Carlisle (Pa.) Hospital
and
Professor of Radiology
Thomas Jefferson University
Philadelphia, Pa.

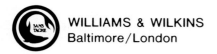
WILLIAMS & WILKINS
Baltimore/London

Reprinted 1979, 1981, 1982, 1984

Made in the United States of America

Library of Congress Cataloging in Publication Data

Harris, John Harold, 1925–
    The radiology of acute cervical spine trauma.

    Includes index.
    1. Vertebrae, Cervical—Wounds and injuries. 2. Vertebrae, Cervical—Radiography. I. Title. [DNLM: 1. Cervical vertebrae—Injuries. 2. Cervical vertebrae—Injuries. 2. Cervical vertebrae—Radiography. We725 H314r]
    RD533.H37   617'.471   78-4112
    ISBN 0-683-03927-X

Composed and printed at the
Waverly Press, Inc.
Mt. Royal and Guilford Aves.
Baltimore, Md. 21202, U.S.A.

DEDICATION

To my sons John and Bob, for reasons best known to them;

to my brother, William H. Harris, M.D., whose uncompromising commitment to excellence is my constant inspiration;

and to my wife, Catherine, whose tolerance, support, and love defy description.

FOREWORD

Having known the author all of his life and having helped train him, I was delighted to be asked to write this foreword. It has given me an opportunity to state publicly what I think of the author. Then, too, he had much to say about the complexities of an extremely common injury. Happily, the work was so thoroughly prepared there was little opportunity for my personal bias to distort my evaluation or appreciation of the text.

The author has made a serious effort to explain the dynamics involved in acute cervical injuries. By so doing and by stressing too the anatomy involved he has given us an authoritative work dealing with acute cervical spine injuries.

One soon appreciates the depth of the author's commitment to his subject. It is clear he feels optimal management of cervical spine injuries is directly related and indeed contingent upon the fidelity of their roentgen demonstration. Using no "gimmickry" he has presented its problems and solutions with consummate clarity. I found some of the going tough for the explanations were not always easy to follow. Nothing remained obscure, however; it merely meant greater concentration on the part of the reader. Unfortunately, the roentgen anatomy of the cervical spine is complex and even under the best circumstances may give one difficulty in its interpretation.

The majority of the illustrations were excellent. Unhappily sometimes it becomes almost an impossibility to obtain optimal radiographic quality in an acute cervical spine problem. Despite an occasional illustration difficulty one leaves the text with a more solid comprehension of "what and why."

To return to the author, Dr. Harris here again demonstrated a clarity of thought and tenacious seeking of the truth that has been his life long habit. Minor details were never given short shrift; nor was he given to over-emphasizing the dramatic.

The work is a balanced presentation of an extremely difficult type of injury. It will stand the test of time for it is an honest appraisal excellently illustrated and not verbose.

PHILIP J. HODES, M.D., D.Sc.
Professor of Radiology
Department of Radiology
University of Miami School of Medicine
P.O. Box 520875
Miami, Florida 33152

PREFACE

The management of acute cervical spine injury begins with the correct roentgen diagnosis of the lesion.

The roentgen diagnosis of acute injuries of the cervical spine depends upon the appropriate radiographic projections obtained in a sequence commensurate with the severity of injury and the clinical condition of the patient. Beyond this, the roentgen diagnosis requires a knowledge of the radiographic anatomy of the cervical spine, particularly its posterior elements, an understanding of the physiology of the normal movements of the cervical spine, and an awareness of the mechanism of injury of the various types of traumatic lesions that may involve the cervical region.

The purpose of this book is to describe and illustrate the radiographic aspects of acute cervical spine trauma. It is readily apparent that there is not a uniformity of opinion in the existing medical literature regarding the etiology and roentgen appearance of all acute injuries of the cervical spine, and it is freely acknowledged that there may be disagreement with some of the content material of this text. However, the concepts presented here do reflect the consensus of an extensive review of the literature relating to acute cervical spine trauma as well as the experienced gained through a broad personal involvement in the roentgen evaluation of patients with acute cervical spine injuries.

This work was born of the frustration engendered by the lack of a ready source of reference for assistance in the evaluation of acute cervical spine injuries as encountered in a busy general practice of radiology. It is designed to ameliorate similar frustrations which might be experienced by other radiologists, orthopedic and neurosurgeons, emergency physicians, and others involved in the diagnosis and management of patients with acute cervical spine injury.

It is sincerely hoped that this effort leads, not only to improved physician knowledge and understanding, but more importantly, to improved patient care.

JHH JR

ACKNOWLEDGMENTS

The production of a textbook requires the interest, effort, and dedication of many people without whose varied contributions the text would never exist.

The mainstay of any diagnostic radiology text is the quality of its illustrations. These begin with the original radiographic examinations. With a single exception, all of the illustrations of this text are the product of roentgen examinations made by the staff and student technologists of the Department of Radiology of the Carlisle Hospital. The quality of the illustrations is a direct measure of the interest and ability of our technologist staff.

The illustrations, themselves, are the result of the combined efforts of the outstanding technical capability of Arrco Medical Art and Photography of Boston, Massachusetts, who produced the negatives, and the dedication and empathy of James Steinmetz of Carlisle, Pennsylvania, who graciously accommodated the author's insistence upon faithful reproduction of the prints.

Jack Edeiken, my close friend, is the person most responsible for the existence of this text. The opportunities and challenges that Dr. Edeiken made possible were the initial stimuli and the sustaining motivation for this work.

Joan Frey Boytim is a multitalented individual who has taken time from her many responsibilities to create the drawings which so richly illustrate important anatomic and radiographic features of cervical spine trauma. The drawings contribute materially to an understanding of the topic.

My associates, Drs. Charles K. Loh, H. C. Perlman, David R. Royal, and Paul T. Collura, have supported and contributed to this work through their interest, enthusiasm, and penetrating questions. Dr. Loh has willingly devoted many hours to a critical review of the manuscript.

The representatives of the Williams & Wilkins Company, particularly Mrs. Ruby Richardson, editor, and Mr. Robert Och, production editor, have exemplified the grace, cordial assistance, and outstanding technical knowledge and ability that are the hallmarks of this distinguished publishing house.

Finally, and as the bedrock of this statement of acknowledgment, it is with greatest pride and highest praise that I freely recognize the invaluable contribution of my secretary, Jane Lendvay Conley, to the successful completion of this manuscript. While calmly, and with gentle good humor, tolerating the effects of the author's biorhythm cycles (which cover a range of approximately 2000 Hounsfield units), and performing the myriad details of a busy department, Mrs. Conley has so thoroughly and efficiently prepared the manuscript that it was submitted to the publisher on schedule without a single error attributable to her work. Mrs. Conley's enthusiasm, loyalty, interest and ability are matchless. It is an absolute fact that without her participation, this book would not exist.

John H. Harris, Jr., M.D.

CONTENTS

CHAPTER 1

THE NORMAL CERVICAL SPINE

I. CHILD

The anatomy of the cervical spine of infants and children that has particular significance for the radiologist relates to ossification of the atlas and axis and hypermobility due to ligamentous laxity, especially the "pseudo-dislocation" at the C_2—C_3 level (1).

Ossification of the atlas begins with the lateral masses during intra-uterine life. At birth, however, neither the anterior nor the posterior arches are fused. During the 2nd year, a center for the posterior tubercle appears and by the end of the 4th year, the posterior arch becomes completely fused.

The anterior arch may fuse from a single center representing the anterior tubercle, multiple centers on each side of the tubercle, or by direct extension from the lateral masses. Fusion is usually complete by the 7th to the 10th year.

While the body of the axis is ossified at birth, the posterior arches are only partially ossified. They fuse, posteriorly, by the 2nd or 3rd year and unite with the body by the 7th year.

The dens ossifies in a cephalad direction, from two centers, which become united at the base of the dens. Distally, a central cleft separates the tips of the ossification centers (Fig. 1.1). A separate ossification center, the ossiculum terminale (Fig. 1.2), is frequently seen in children and may persist as late as the 11th year.

The dens is separated from the body of the axis, normally, by a broad cartilagenous band corresponding to an intervertebral disk. This "sub-

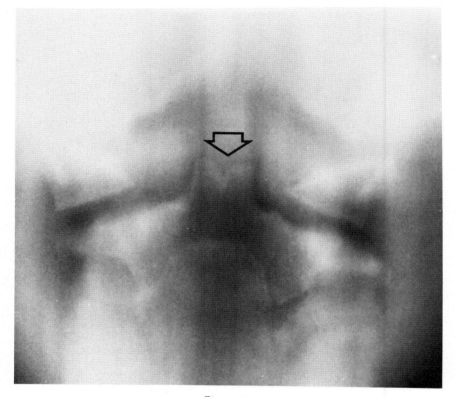

Figure 1.1
Normal appearance of the dens in a young child demonstrating the cleft between the tips of the ossification centers of the body of the dens (arrow).

chondral synchondrosis" is present in all children to the age of 3 years (Fig. 1.3). It gradually decreases in width, but may persist as a thin radiolucent stripe with densely sclerotic margins until early adolescence. As such, the synchondrosis may simulate a fracture (Fig. 1.4).

In infants and young children, normal laxity of the soft tissues of the cervico-cranium may result in perplexing shadows on the lateral radiograph of the cervical spine.

Physiologic laxity of the retropharyngeal prevertebral soft tissues may simulate a retropharyngeal tumor, abscess, or hematoma unless great care is taken to obtain the lateral radiograph of the neck in extension and during maximum inspiration (Fig. 1.5, a and b).

Physiologic range of motion at the atlanto-axial level during flexion and extension is greater in infants and children than in adults. The atlanto-dental interval (ADI), because of looseness of the capsules and ligaments, may range from 2 to 5 mm, with the maximum ADI occurring

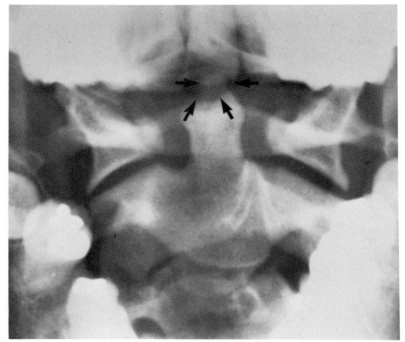

Figure 1.2
Ossiculum terminale (arrows).

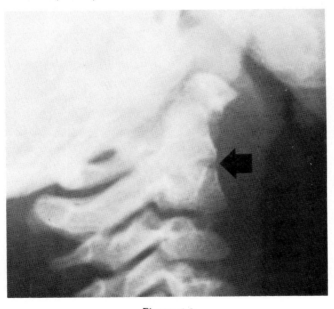

Figure 1.3
The subchondral synchondrosis, between the dens and the body of the axis (arrow), is normally present to age 3 years.

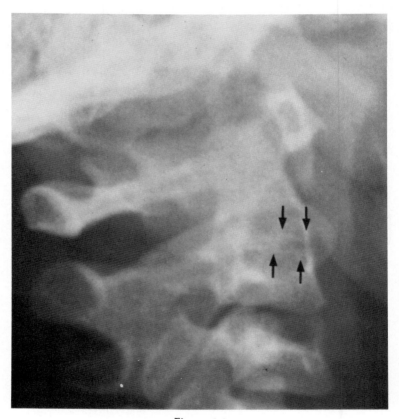

Figure 1.4
Faintly sclerotic margins (arrow) mark the residuum of a fused subchondral synchondrosis.

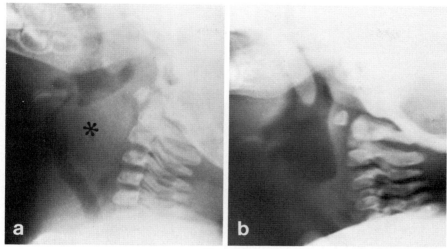

Figure 1.5
The effect of inspiration and positioning on the retropharyngeal soft tissues of an infant. (a) Exposure made during expiration and without cervical extension demonstrates a large retropharyngeal pseudo-mass (*). (b) Same patient, minutes later. Radiograph obtained during inspiration and with gentle cervical extension.

in flexion (2) (Fig. 1.6). The ADI most frequently measures 2mm and, according to a study by Locke *et al.* (3), in 92–97% of 200 children did not exceed 3 mm.

Cattell and Filtzer (4) have noted that in 20% of normal children under 8 years of age, more than two-thirds of the anterior arch of the atlas lay above the tip of the dens in extension (Fig. 1.7).

"Pseudo-subluxation" and "pseudo-dislocation" are terms applied to the anterior displacement of C_2 on C_3 frequently seen in infants and young children. Physiologic anterior displacement of C_2 on C_3 occurs in 24% of children under the age of 8 years. A lesser incidence (14%) of pseudo-dislocation may occur at the C_3–C_4 level (4). The mobility of these cervical segments has been attributed to the normal laxity of the ligaments of the cervical spine during childhood, to the shallow angle of the apophyseal joints at these levels, and to the fact that the C_2–C_3 level, which is the site of transition between the cervico-cranium and the lower cervical segments, acts as the fulcrum for flexion and extension (5, 6).

The physiologic anterior displacement of C_2 on C_3 is frequently difficult to distinguish from pathologic displacement, particularly in a patient with a history of cervical trauma. Swischuk (6) has described the "posterior cervical line" (Fig. 1.8) and its relationship to the anterior

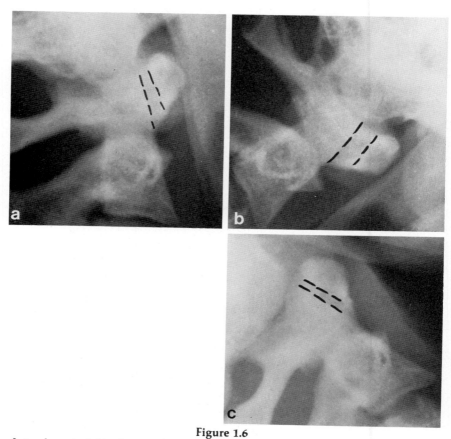

Figure 1.6
Lateral neutral (a), flexion (b), and extension (c) radiographs of the atlanto-axial articulation in a normal 5-year-old boy. The width of the space between the arch of C_1 and the dens (ADI) measured 3 mm in neutral, 5mm in flexion, and 2mm in extension.

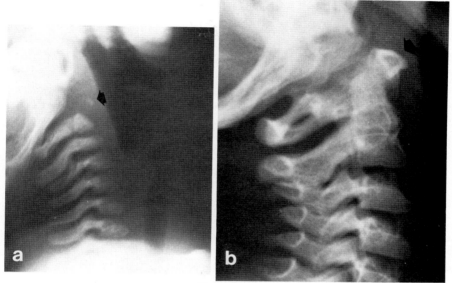

Figure 1.7
Normal relationship of the anterior arch of the atlas and the dens in extension. (a) Infant. (b) Young child. ([b] Reprinted by permission from Harris, J. H. Jr. & Harris, W. H.: *The Radiology of Emergency Medicine.* Williams & Wilkins, Baltimore, Md. © 1975.)

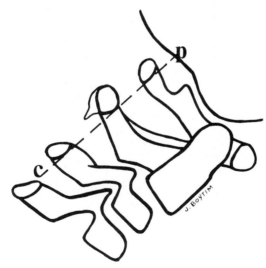

Figure 1.8
Schematic representation of posterior cervical line (pc).

cortex of the spinous process of C_2 as indicating whether displacement of C_2 is physiologic or due to a fracture-dislocation of C_2.

The posterior cervical line is a line extending from the anterior cortex of the posterior arch of the atlas to the anterior cortex of the posterior arch of C_3. Normally, the anterior cortex of the posterior arch of C_2 lies posterior to the posterior cervical line in extension and neutral positions. In pseudo-subluxation of C_2, where the entire vertebra is anteriorly displaced, the posterior cervical line may: *(a)* touch the anterior cortex of the posterior arch of C_2 (Fig. 1.9); *(b)* pass through the anterior cortex;

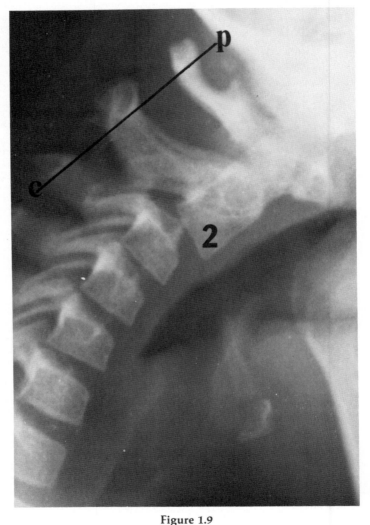

Figure 1.9
Pseudo-subluxation of C_2 on C_3. The anterior cortical surface of the posterior arch of C_2 touches the posterior cervical line (pc).

or *(c)* lie 1.5–2.0 mm anterior to the anterior cortex of the posterior arch of C_2. This relationship obtains even when the body of C_2 is displaced forward with respect to that of C_3. If the anterior cortex of the neural arch of C_2 lies more than 2 mm behind the posterior cervical line, a bilateral fracture of its neural arch (hangman's fracture) may be presumed.

II. ADULT

A. Cervico-cranium

The anatomy of the cervical spine begins with the occiput and the occipital condyles. The occiput, the atlas, and the axis, when considered as a unit, are referred to as the "cervico-cranium" (7). This designation is warranted by the distinctive anatomy of this region which clearly differs from that of the majority of the cervical spine. The effects of trauma to this segment of the central axis are reflective of these unique structural characteristics.

The atlanto-occipital joints are formed by the convex articulating surface of the occipital condyles and the concave superior surface of the lateral masses of the atlas.

The ligaments connecting the occiput and atlas include the thin

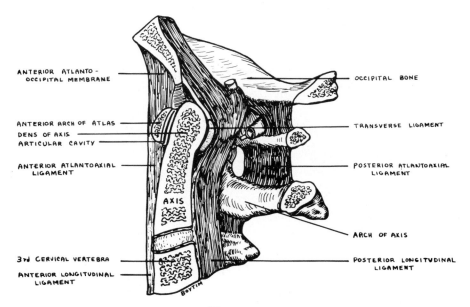

Figure 1.10

Schematic sagittal representation of the cervico-cranium. (Reprinted by permission from Harris, J. H. Jr. & Harris, W. H.: *The Radiology of Emergency Medicine*. Williams & Wilkins, Baltimore, Md. © 1975.)

articular capsules, the broad, dense anterior atlanto-occipital ligament (membrane) which extends from the anterior margin of the foramen magnum to the cranial aspect of the anterior arch of the atlas, the broad posterior atlanto-occipital ligament which passes from the posterior margin of the foramen magnum to the superior margin of the posterior arch of the atlas, and the dense, thin lateral atlanto-occipital ligaments which extend from the occipital bone to the transverse process of the atlas (Fig. 1.10 and 1.11).

The first cervical segment, the atlas (Fig. 1.12), is a unique ring-like

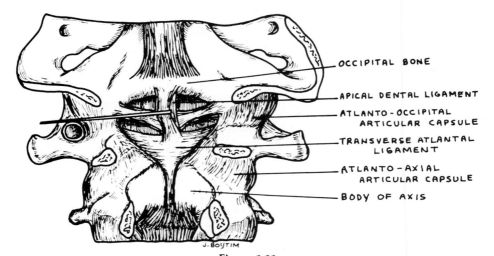

Figure 1.11
Major ligamentous structures of the cervico-cranium, seen from behind.

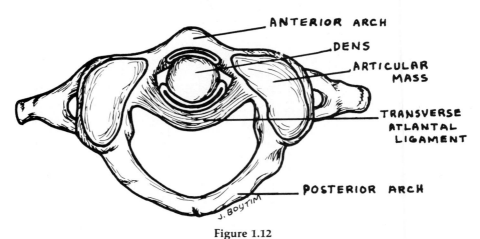

Figure 1.12
The atlas seen from above. Note the position of the transverse atlantal ligament to the dens.

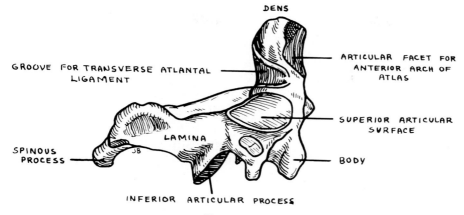

DENS

ARTICULAR FACET FOR
ANTERIOR ARCH OF
ATLAS

GROOVE FOR TRANSVERSE ATLANTAL
LIGAMENT

SUPERIOR ARTICULAR
SURFACE

LAMINA

SPINOUS
PROCESS

BODY

INFERIOR ARTICULAR PROCESS

Figure 1.13

The axis seen in lateral projection. Note that the convex superior facet is horizontally situated while the inferior facet is obliquely anteriorly and inferiorly oriented to form the superior component of the highest interfacetal joint. (Reprinted by permission from Harris, J. H. Jr. & Harris, W. H.: *The Radiology of Emergency Medicine*. Williams & Wilkins, Baltimore, Md. © 1975. After Figure 4.16, *Gray's Anatomy*.)

vertebra characterized by the absence of a vertebral body. It consists of an anterior arch, a lateral mass on each side, and a posterior arch. It does not contain pedicles or laminae, as do other cervical vertebrae, and has no true spinous process. The anterior and posterior arches are relatively thin. The lateral masses, cn the other hand, are heavy, thick structures. Each has a concave superior and a convex inferior articulating surface. A rudimentary transverse process extends laterally from each mass and contains the transverse foramen through which passes the vertebral artery.

The short, dense, thick transverse atlantal ligament extends between the medial surfaces of the lateral masses (Fig. 1.12) and maintains the normal relationship of the dens to the anterior arch of C_1.

The second cervical vertebra, the axis, is the largest and heaviest of the cervical segments (Fig. 1.13). Like the remainder of the cervical vertebrae, it consists of a body, bilateral masses (articular masses, "pillars"), laminae, and a thick heavy spinous process. It is unique by virtue of the odontoid process (dens), which arises from multiple ossification centers, creating an upward extension of the body of the axis and which serves as the pivotal point of atlantal rotation. The superior articulating facets of the axis are convex, while the inferior facets face obliquely forward and downward.

The atlas and axis articulate through four joints, the median and the bilateral atlanto-axial joints (8). The articulation between the posterior surface of the anterior arch of C_1 and the anterior surface of the dens and that between the posterior surface of the dens and the transverse atlantal ligament, together, constitute the median atlanto-axial (pivot) joint. Each of these components has a true, separate, synovial joint space (Figs. 1.10 and 1.12).

The lateral atlanto-axial joints are formed by the contiguous articulating surfaces of the lateral masses of the atlas and axis. These joints are arthrodial and each articulating surface of each joint is convex. In the neutral position, therefore, the articulating surfaces of the atlas and axis are in contact at the highest points of their convex surfaces. During rotation, the inferior facets of the atlas, moving either anteriorly or posteriorly, come to be in contact with the superior facet of the axis at some point lower than the apex of its convex surface. This has been referred to as "telescoping" (9) and is the explanation for "vertical approximation," the term used by Hohl (10) to describe the apparent decrease in combined vertical height of the atlas and axis in extreme rotation.

The roentgen appearance of the cervico-cranium in frontal projection, *i.e.*, the "open-mouth" view, is seen in Figure 1.14. The important observations are that the atlas sits squarely upon the axis with the dens equidistant between the lateral masses of the atlas, that the lateral atlanto-axial joint spaces are open and their contiguous surfaces parallel, that the lateral margins of the lateral atlanto-axial surfaces are precisely superimposed and symmetrical, and that the bifid spinous process of the axis is in the midline.

The principal ligament at the atlanto-axial articulation is the transverse atlantal ligament. Other ligaments which contribute to the function of the atlanto-axial articulation include the alar, the apical odontoid, and the cruciate ligaments. The alar ("check") ligaments, which arise from each side of the dens and pass laterally to the medial surface of each occipital condyle (Fig. 1.11), limit rotation and participate in preventing anterior atlantal subluxation (11). The apical odontoid ligament is a slender band that extends from the tip of the dens to the anterior rim of the foramen magnum. The cruciate ligaments are small bands of fiber that arise from the posterior surface of the middle of the transverse ligament and extend upward to the anterior rim of the foramen magnum and downward to the axis. These ligaments are involved in maintaining the normal relationship of the cervico-cranium and in the complex motions at the C_1–C_2 level (Fig. 1.11).

The anterior atlanto-axial ligament (Fig. 1.10) is the upward extension of the anterior longitudinal ligament. The posterior longitudinal ligament extends from the basilar portion of the occiput, posterior to the

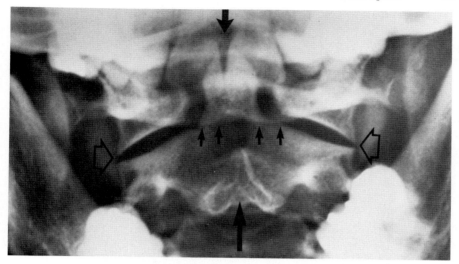

Figure 1.14

The atlanto-axial articulation seen in the open-mouth view. The dens is centrally located between the lateral masses of the axis, the lateral margins of the lateral atlanto-axial joints are precisely symmetrical (open arrows), and the spinous process of C_2 (stemmed arrow) is in the midline. Two frequently perplexing natural artifacts are illustrated. The space between the central maxillary incisor teeth (large arrow) simulates a vertical defect in the dens. The thin, curvilinear, transverse lucent band at the base of the dens (small arrows) is caused by the Mach effect of the superimposed anterior arch of the atlas. This may be mistaken for a fracture line. (Reprinted by permission from Harris, J. H. Jr.: Acute injuries of the spine. *Semin. Roentgenol.* 13:53, 1978.)

dens and its ligamentous complex, to the posterior surface of the axis and from there downward as the anterior surface of the neural canal.

The lateral radiographic appearance of the cervico-cranium of a normal adult is seen in Figure 1.15. It is important to be aware that air in the pharynx outlines the soft palate and uvula, the base of the tongue and the naso-oro-pharyngeal airway. The shadow representing the normal soft tissue structures of the naso-oro-pharynx is closely adherent to the anterior surface of the atlas and axis and extends upward to the clivus and inferiorly to be continuous with the soft tissues of the posterior wall of the hypopharynx. Above the level of the anterior arch of the atlas, this soft tissue shadow represents principally the anterior atlanto-occipital ligament and from the anterior inferior corner of the axis to the atlas, principally the anterior atlanto-axial ligament which is, in effect, the cephalic extension of the anterior longitudinal ligament.

The normal relationship between the posterior surface of the anterior arch of the atlas and the anterior surface of the dens (atlanto-dental

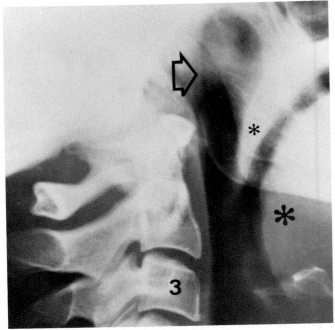

Figure 1.15
Lateral radiograph of the upper cervical spine of a normal adult. The soft palate and uvula (small asterisk) and the base of the tongue (large asterisk) are delineated by air in the naso-oro-pharynx. The posterior wall of the nasopharynx, formed principally by the atlanto-occipital ligament, is indicated by the open arrow. The soft tissues of the posterior pharyngeal wall are closely adherent to the anterior surfaces of the second and third vertebrae. The soft tissue shadow anterior to the body of C₃ does not normally exceed 4 mm in the adult. (Reprinted by permission from Harris, J. H. Jr.: The significance of soft tissue injury in the roentgen diagnosis of trauma. *CRC Crit. Rev. Clin. Radiol. Nucl. Med.* 295, July, 1975.) Copyright the Chemical Rubber Co., CRC Press, Inc.

interval, ADI) is maintained by the transverse atlantal ligament and does not normally exceed 3 mm in adults, in neutral, flexion, and extension positions (11, 12) (Fig. 1.16).

The posterior arch of the atlas is small compared to the size of the occiput and the heavy spinous process of the axis. The posterior arches of C_1 should, in a properly positioned lateral radiograph, be superimposed upon each other with a distinct soft tissue space between the posterior ring of C_1 and the occiput, above, and the laminae and spinous process of the axis, below. The width of these spaces, especially the occipito-atlantal space, varies with flexion and extension (Fig. 1.16).

B. Lower Cervical Vertebrae

The third through the seventh cervical vertebrae are identical in shape, but increase gradually in size with the seventh being the largest and heaviest of these. Transverse processes extend laterally from the vertebral body. They are concave superiorly and carry the cervical roots as they leave the neural canal.

The contiguous articulating facets of the lateral masses from C_2 through C_7 comprise the interfacetal (facetal, apophyseal) joints. The inferior facet of the vertebra above constitutes the superior facet of the joint and the superior articulating facet of the vertebra below constitutes the inferior facet of the joint. The inferior facet of the vertebra above is directed anteriorly and inferiorly, while the superior facet of the subjacent vertebra is oriented posteriorly and superiorly. The plane of the

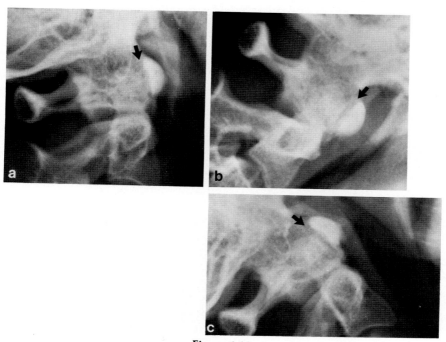

Figure 1.16

The normal relationship of the atlas and axis in lateral neutral (a), flexion (b), and extension (c). The distance between the posterior surface of the anterior arch of the atlas and the anterior surface of the dens (atlanto-dental-interval, ADI) (arrow) does not normally exceed 3 mm in the adult. (Reprinted by permission from Harris, J. H. Jr. & Harris, W. H.: *The Radiology of Emergency Medicine.* Williams & Wilkins, Baltimore, Md. © 1975.)

interfacetal joints is angled approximately 35° posteriorly from the vertical. For purposes of clarity, consistency, and simplicity of expression, the articulating facets will, in all subsequent discussions, be defined as they comprise the interfacetal joint, *i.e.*, the superior facet (of the joint) and the inferior facet (of the joint).

The superior facet is normally situated above and behind the inferior facet. The posterior margins of the articulating facets are closely parallel and symmetrical in the neutral position (Fig. 1.17).

Soft tissue structures with less specific functions than those previously

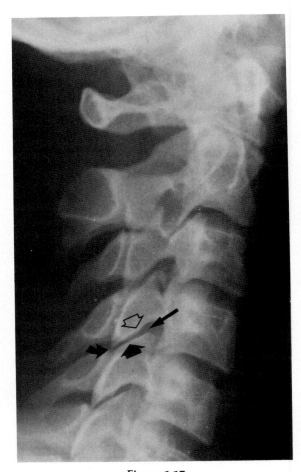

Figure 1.17
Lateral radiograph of a normal adult cervical spine demonstrating an interfacetal joint (stemmed arrow) and its superior (open arrow) and inferior (solid arrow) facets. The posterior margins of the contiguous articulating facets are closely parallel (curved arrow).

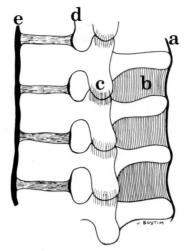

Figure 1.18

Schematic representation of the major ligaments of the lower cervical spine; (a) represents the supraspinous ligament, (b) the interspinous ligament, (c) the articular capsule of an interfacetal joint, (d) the posterior longitudinal ligament, and (e) the anterior longitudinal ligament. (Reprinted by permission from Harris, J. H. Jr.: Acute injuries of the spine. *Semin. Roentgenol.* 13:53, 1978.)

described are present throughout the cervical area and are important to cervical stability and motion.

The supraspinous ligament (Fig. 1.18a) is a strong fibrous cord that connects the apices of the spinous processes from the external occipital protuberance to the sacrum. The ligamentum nuchae is that segment of the supraspinous ligament which extends from the spinous process of C_7 to the external occipital protuberance. A fibrous membrane penetrates from the ligamentum nuchae deep into the neck to attach onto the spinous process of the cervical segments, thereby forming a septum between the muscles on each side of the posterior aspect of the neck.

The interspinous ligaments (Fig. 1.18b) are thin membranous structures which connect adjacent spinous processes. They extend from the base to the tip of each spinous process.

The thin, loose capsules of the interfacetal joints (Fig. 1.18c) attach to the margins of the articular surfaces of the adjacent vertebrae.

The ligamentum flava (Fig. 1.19) are thick, dense, broad structures that connect the laminae of adjacent vertebrae. These ligaments arise from the ventral surface of the lamina above and pass inferiorly to attach to the dorsal surface of the lamina below where the laminae fuse to form the base of the spinous process.

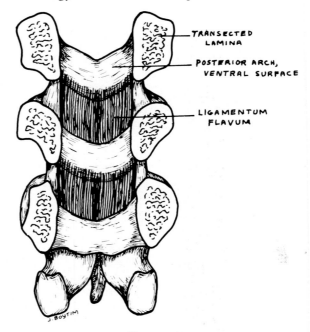

Figure 1.19
Schematic representation of the ventral aspect of the posterior neural arch. Note that the ligamenta flava arise from the ventral surface of the lamina above and insert on the posterior surface of the lamina below.

The posterior longitudinal ligament (Fig. 1.18d) extends from the axis to the sacrum. It is a dense broad ligament lying within the ventral surface of the spinal canal, closely adherent to the posterior surface of the vertebral bodies and disks.

The intervertebral disks (Fig. 1.18), being interposed between the contiguous surfaces of adjacent vertebrae, constitute the chief connection between the vertebral bodies. They are closely adherent to the anterior and posterior longitudinal ligaments.

The dense, strong anterior longitudinal ligament (Fig. 1.18e) extends from the anterior inferior surface of the axis (C_2) to the sacrum. It is closely adherent to the intervertebral disks and the prominent margins of the vertebrae, but is not tightly adherent to the concavity of the anterior surfaces of the vertebral bodies.

The antero-posterior radiograph of the cervical spine of a normal adult is seen in Figure 1.20. Because of the density caused by superimposition of the mandible and occiput, the atlanto-axial articulation cannot be seen in this projection. The lower five cervical and upper thoracic segments are recorded in anterior view. The superior and inferior end-plates, the lateral cortical margins, and the uncinate processes of the vertebral bodies, as well as the joints of Luschka are usually clearly recorded in this projection. The interfacetal joint spaces, which are angled postero-inferiorly approximately 35°, cannot be seen in this projection because of the superimposition of the lateral masses. As a result of the superimposition, the lateral cortical margins of the articular masses appear as a continuous, smoothly undulating, sharply defined density at the lateral edges of the cervical spine. The spinous processes are in the midline. The margins of the air shadow in the upper trachea and subglottic area are tapered symmetrically toward the midline.

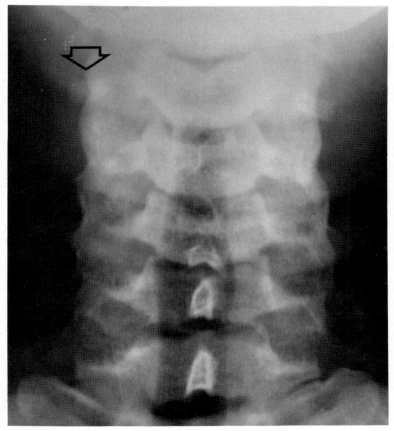

Figure 1.20
Antero-posterior radiograph of the normal adult cervical spine. The spinous processes are in the midline. The lateral margins of the articular masses, because of their superimposition in this projection, appear as a continuous, smoothly undulating cortical density (arrow).

In contradistinction to the frontal radiograph, the lateral projection of the cervical spine (Fig. 1.21) does include the atlas and axis. The vertebrae are normally aligned in a gentle, smooth lordotic curve. The vertebral bodies may be nearly square or slightly rectangular in the antero-posterior dimension. The contiguous surfaces of the disk spaces are normally parallel. This may be modified by anomalies of the cervical vertebrae or either localized or diffuse osteoarthritis. The transverse processes are superimposed upon the vertebral bodies and the pedicles. The pedicles are commonly not visualized because of their shortness and the superimposed transverse processes.

Positioning for the lateral radiograph is critical in order that the lateral masses be so precisely superimposed that, even though they are paired structures, they appear as one with a single posterior cortical line. The articulating surfaces (facets) of the interfacetal joints should be super-imposed so that it appears as though there is a single interfacetal joint space at each level. The posterior margins of the articulating facets of the apophyseal joints are closely superimposed. From the level of the third spinous process downward, the interspinous spaces are of approximately the same height. The second interspinous space is commonly greater than the others.

Even slight rotation causes anterior displacement of the articular masses of one side with respect to those of the opposite side. Radiographically, this is evident by the lack of superimposition of the posterior cortical margins of the masses and of the interfacetal joints. If the entire spine is rotated uniformly, the amount of asymmetry of the posterior cortices of the lateral masses will be the same throughout the cervical area (Fig. 1.22). Improper positioning for the lateral radiograph characterized by simple rotation of the head with respect to the cervical spine results in gradually increasing amounts of asymmetry of the lateral masses from the lower to the upper cervical segments (Fig. 1.23).

It is important to be aware of the effect of these two types of improper positioning upon the lateral radiograph of the cervical spine so that they not be misinterpreted as the rotational component of unilateral interfacetal dislocation.

The width of the soft tissue shadow anterior to the body of C_3 is an important landmark. Hay (13) has developed a formula by which the normal width of this soft tissue shadow can be calculated, based upon patient age. Practically, however, the width of the soft tissue density anterior to the body of C_3 does not normally exceed 4 mm in adults (Fig. 1.15).

Flexion and extension occur in a gradual, sequential fashion with the amount of motion being greatest at the upper levels (Fig. 1.24). Fielding

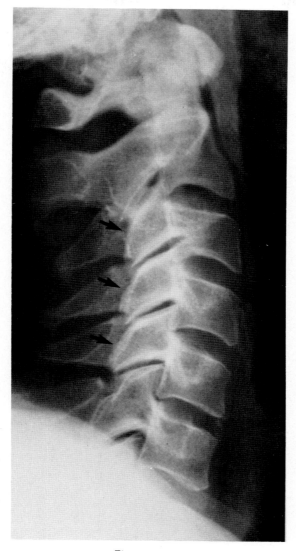

Figure 1.21

Lateral radiograph of a normal adult cervical spine. The vertebrae are aligned in a gentle lordotic configuration. The posterior margins of the vertebral bodies constitute a continous concave sweep, while the curve of the anterior surface is convex. The lateral (articular) masses are superimposed and so, consequently, are the interfacetal joint spaces and their superior and inferior articulating facets. The paired posterior cortical surfaces of the lateral masses (arrows) are superimposed and appear as a single cortical density.

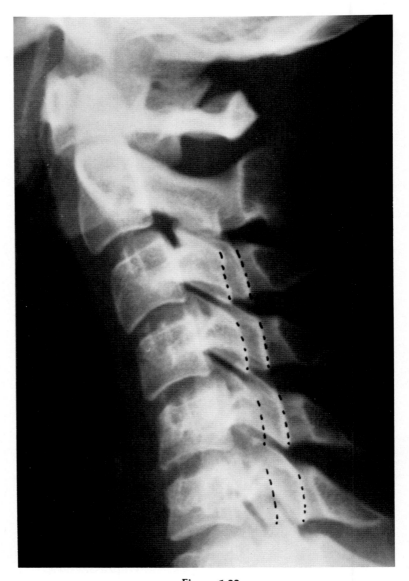

Figure 1.22
With the entire body rotated slightly forward on its central axis, the articular masses are no longer superimposed. The posterior cortical surfaces (broken lines) of one side lie anterior to those of the opposite side. The degree of lack of superimposition is similar at each level because the entire cervical spine has rotated as a unit.

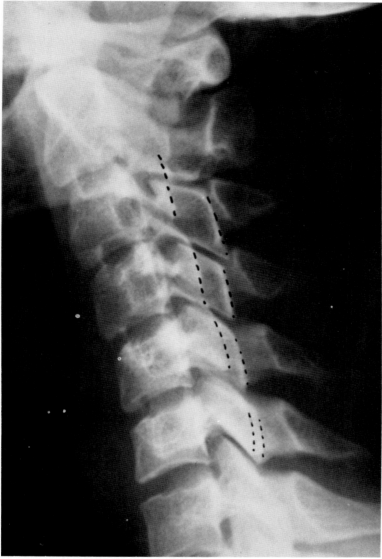

Figure 1.23

Improper positioning caused by rotation of the head alone. In this example, the body is in lateral position relative to its central axis, but the head has been allowed to rotate slightly. Because rotation of the head involves primarily the atlas and axis, there is progressively greater lack of superimposition of the articular masses from the lower through the upper segments.

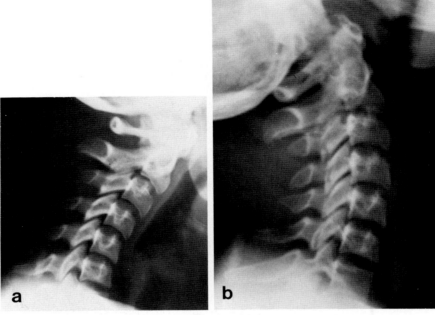

Figure 1.24
Lateral radiograph of a normal adult cervical spine in flexion (a). Each successively higher segment pivots and glides slightly more forward than the segment below. Movement is greatest at the higher levels. This results in a uniform reversal of the normal cervical lordotic curve. All of the interspaces are narrowed anteriorly and widened posteriorly. The superior facets glide forward on the inferior facets and the interspinous spaces widen. In extension (b), all of the changes of flexion are reversed.

(14) states, "Below the second cervical vertebra, motion at one interspace gradually does not occur without similar motion taking place at other levels." During flexion (Fig. 1.24a), there is a continuum of movement from the lower through the upper segments, characterized by each segment gliding forward and pivoting on its anterior inferior corner. As a result the continuous curve projected by the posterior surfaces of the vertebral bodies becomes smoothly convex throughout the cervical spine and the curve of the anterior surfaces, concave. The intervertebral spaces become slightly narrowed anteriorly and widened posteriorly as the disk is compressed anteriorly by the movement of the vertebral bodies. The articular masses glide upward and forward in gradually increasing, but related distances from the seventh to the second segment. The interspinous spaces, from the seventh through the third, increase uniformly in width.

These movements are reversed in extension (Fig. 1.24b).

The oblique radiograph of the cervical spine is made with the patient approximately 45° off of the frontal (or lateral) position. In positioning the patient for the oblique projection, it is important that the entire patient be rotated about the longitudinal axis of the spine rather than simply rotating the head and neck. A properly positioned oblique radiograph of a normal adult spine is seen in Figure 1.25.

The purpose of this examination is to visualize the pedicles, the intervertebral foramina, the lateral masses, and the interfacetal joints. In a properly positioned oblique view, the central beam passes directly through the intervertebral foramina, clearly delineating the foramina and their margins. The transverse processes are superimposed upon the pedicles. Normally, depending upon anatomic variations of the transverse processes or minor deviations from the true oblique position, the transverse processes may be projected into the foramina. The normal

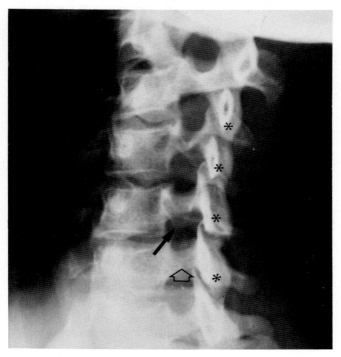

Figure 1.25

Oblique radiograph of the normal cervical spine. The superior facets of the joint (*) are posterior to the inferior facets. The intervertebral foramina are all open. The pedicles (open arrow) connecting the vertebral bodies and the articular masses are clearly demonstrated. A transverse process may be superimposed upon a foramen (stemmed arrow).

relationship of the superior facet above and posterior to the inferior facet (of the joint) is well illustrated in oblique projection. The configuration of the articular masses varies with minor alterations of positioning (Fig. 1.26, a and b). The articular masses and interfacetal joints of the opposite side are not well seen because they are superimposed upon the vertebral bodies, hence each oblique radiograph is required to evaluate the posterior elements completely.

The pillar (Weir [15]) view (Fig. 1.27) is designed to demonstrate the individual lateral masses in the coronal plane. This projection is particularly important in the detection of acute fractures of the lateral mass. The pillar view is made with the patient supine and the head in

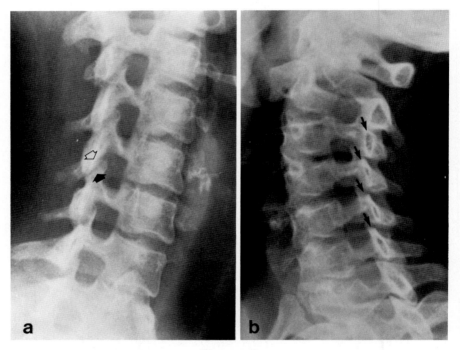

Figure 1.26
Minor variations in obliquity result in minor differences in the roentgen appearance of the articular masses and their facets. In (a), the normal relationship of the superior facet (open arrow) to the inferior facet (solid arrow) of the joint is clearly evident. In (b), however, the articular masses and facets are not well visualized. Instead, the laminae are seen "end-on" as obliquely situated structures with cortical margins (arrows). Although the articulating facets are not clearly defined, the laminae have the same anatomic relationship to each other as do the lateral masses, *i.e.,* the lamina of the vertebra above is posterior and superior to the lamina of the vertebra below. Therefore, in an oblique projection such as this, the laminae indicate the normal alignment of the posterior elements of the cervical vertebrae.

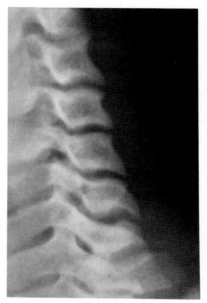

Figure 1.27
Normal pillar (Weir) view of the left articular masses.

maximum rotation to eliminate superimposition of the mandible and face upon the lateral masses of the side being examined. The x-ray tube is angled 35° caudad with the central beam off-centered 2 cm from the midline in the direction opposite that to which the head is rotated. The central beam is centered at the level of the thyroid cartilage. If possible, depending upon the condition of the patient, the lateral masses of the opposite side should be examined by simply reversing the rotation of the head and centering the tube. An alternative method of obtaining a satisfactory pillar view has been suggested by Edeiken (16) when the patient is unable to rotate the head. Under these conditions, the examination is made with the patient erect and with the central beam directed postero-anterior, angled *cephalad* approximately 35°, and centered just above the seventh spinous process.

CHAPTER 2

ROENTGEN EXAMINATION

The roentgen examination of a patient with an acute cervical spine injury is determined by the patient's clinical findings and the description of the injuring incident.

The single most important radiographic study of the acutely, severely injured patient is the horizontal-beam lateral radiograph of the cervical area. "Severely injured" shall include the patient who has one or more of the following: clinical evidence of major injury to the head or neck, who is unconscious, paralyzed, or who has sustained fractures of multiple long bones, or injury to multiple organ systems. In such patients, the horizontal-beam lateral radiograph of the cervical area should be obtained immediately following the institution of resuscitative procedures and before the patient is moved from the litter.

Commonly, the lower cervical segments are obscured by the super-imposed density of the shoulders. Every reasonable effort, consonant with the patient's condition, should be expended to visualize these segments. Usually, gentle traction upon the patient's wrists over a few-minute interval will pull the shoulders sufficiently caudad to expose the lower vertebrae (Fig. 2.1). If not, it is possible to evaluate the lower cervical segments by means of oblique projections obtained with the patient recumbent. By this technique a film is placed as far as possible posterior to the neck. The x-ray tube is off-centered to the opposite side of the neck and angled approximately 45° toward the film and centered to the posterior inferior margin of the thyroid cartilage (Fig. 2.2). The resultant oblique roentgenograms provide useful visualization of the

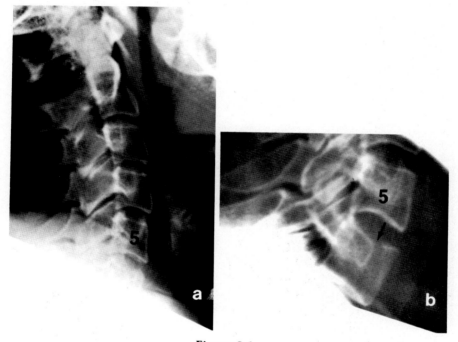

Figure 2.1
In the initial horizontal-beam lateral radiograph (a), the lower segments are obscured by the superimposed density of the shoulders. The shoulders were pulled caudad by gentle sustained traction to the arms, and the subsequent lateral radiograph (b) demonstrated a fracture of C_6.

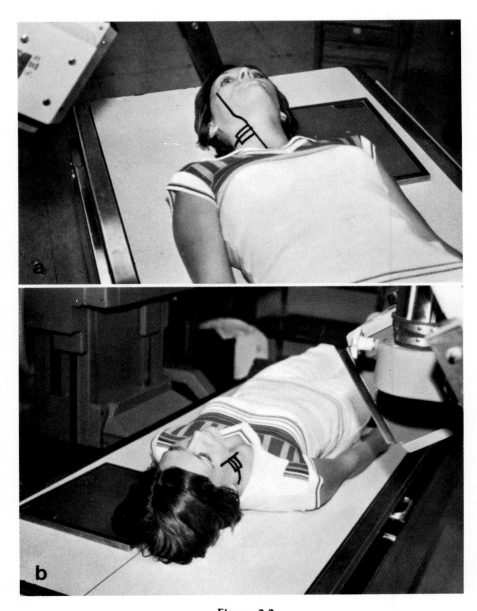

Figure 2.2

Illustrations of positioning for supine oblique projection of the cervical spine.

vertebral bodies, the pedicles, intervertebral foramina, and the articular masses (Fig. 2.3).

In the less severely injured patient, a definite sequence of roentgen examinations (the "basic" examination of the cervical spine) must be

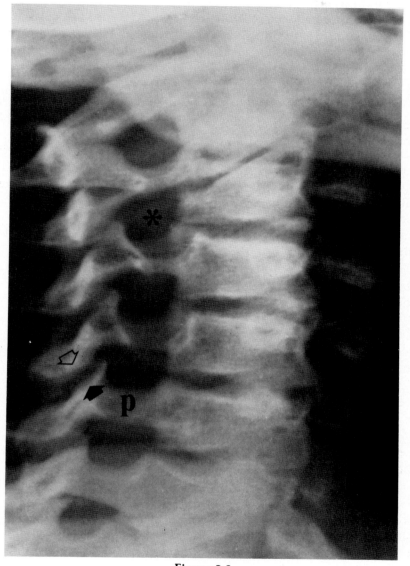

Figure 2.3
Supine oblique radiograph. The postero-lateral aspect of the vertebral bodies, the pedicles (p), the intervertebral foramina (*), and the interfacetal joints (superior facet, open arrow; inferior facet, solid arrow) are clearly delineated.

followed in order to preclude aggravating an existing injury. The sequence must include the antero-posterior projection, the open-mouth view of the atlanto-axial articulation, the lateral radiograph in neutral position, and each oblique projection. These studies must be interpreted by the radiologist before any additional views are obtained. If the basic examination is negative or equivocal, or if the mechanism of injury and the physical findings suggest a subluxation of the cervical spine, then, and only then, are lateral flexion and extension views indicated. A physician should personally supervise positioning of the head and neck in the flexed and extended positions to insure that excessive flexion and extension are not forced.

When the basic examination provides a definitive diagnosis or demonstrates an unstable injury, lateral flexion and extension views are specifically contraindicated.

If the basic study suggests a fracture of the articular mass, the pillar view (15, 17, 18) is usually required to confirm the diagnosis. Tomograms of the lateral masses of the injured side made with the head rotated as far as possible to the opposite side are also valuable in delineating the extent of pillar fractures.

Laminograms, either in frontal or lateral position, are useful in evaluating the integrity of the posterior elements.

Fluoroscopic examination, particularly of unilateral and bilateral interfacetal dislocations, following orthopedic immobilization, is extremely helpful in determining the extent and characteristics of the injury.

Computed tomography (CT) provides excellent demonstration of the cervical spine in axial section. In order to achieve optimum demonstration of the upper cervical segments, precise positioning is required. Not only must rotation be eliminated as much as possible (Fig. 2.4), but the upper portion of the cervical lordosis should be obliterated as well. This can be accomplished by the very careful insertion of a shallow firm wedge posterior to the cervical spine and occiput. This positioning, and the subsequent CT examination, must be personally supervised by the radiologist.

Figure 2.4

Axial tomograms of the atlas, made at 1-cm intervals. The dens (*) is midway between the lateral masses of the atlas (l) (r). Minor imprecision in positioning resulted in the left transverse process being outside the plane of the more cephalad slice (a), and the right transverse process being outside the plane of the next lower slice (b). This emphasizes the importance of meticulous attention to positioning in the CT examination of the cervical spine. (Picker Synerview. Window settings adjusted for the skeleton.)

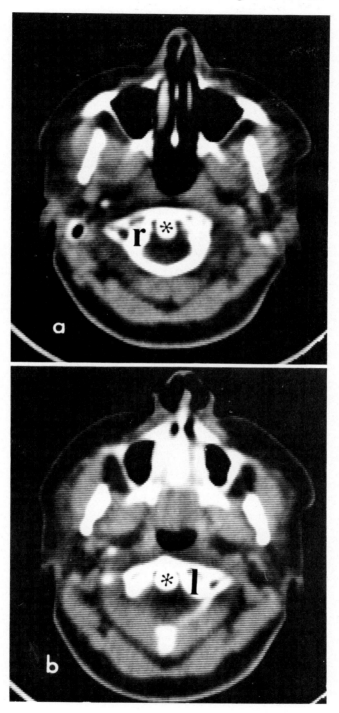

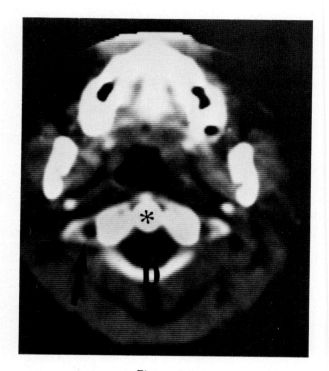

Figure 2.5
Axial tomograph through the atlas. The dens (*) is symmetrically situated between the lateral masses of the atlas. The transverse process of the atlas (stemmed arrow) contains the foramen for the transmission of the vertebral artery. The posterior arch of the atlas is indicated by (p). (Picker Synerview. Window settings adjusted for the skeleton)

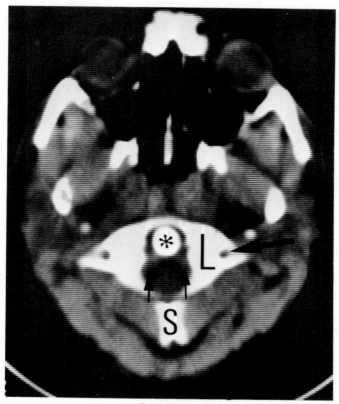

Figure 2.6

Same patient as Figure 2.5. This axial tomograph was made at a 1-cm more cephalad level. The true joint space between the dens (*) and the anterior arch of the atlas is evident. The transverse ligament is indicated by the small stemmed arrows. The lateral masses of the atlas (L) contain the vertebral artery foramen (large stemmed arrow). (S) represents the spinous process of the axis. (Picker Synerview. Window settings adjusted for the skeleton.)

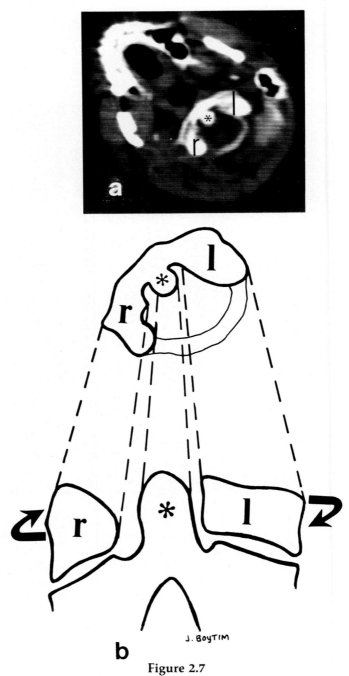

Figure 2.7
CT scan of the normal atlanto-axial articulation made with the head rotated
to the right (a). The left lateral mass of the atlas (l) has rotated anteriorly and

The anatomy of the atlas is clearly demonstrated by axial tomography. The anterior arch, the lateral masses, transverse processes including the vertebral artery foramen, and the posterior arch are all sharply delineated. The relationship of the dens to the anterior arch of the atlas is well demonstrated (Fig. 2.5).

Appropriate utilization of window settings makes visualization of the transverse atlantal ligament and the true joint space between the dens and the anterior arch of the atlas possible (Fig. 2.6).

The effect of rotation of the head upon the atlanto-axial relationship is also clearly demonstrated by computed axial tomography. When viewed from the axial perspective (Fig. 2.7a), the effect of rotation upon the configuration of the lateral masses of C_1, as recorded in the open-mouth projection, is clearly evident (Fig. 2.7b).

Fractures of the dens may be better demonstrated by xerography and rectilinear tomography than by routine radiographic projections.

---

the right lateral mass (r) posteriorly. The schematic representation of the correlation between the axial tomograph of the atlas in rotation and the appearance of the atlas and axis in rotation, as seen in the open-mouth projection, is presented in (b). The anteriorly rotated lateral mass increases in width and the space between it and the dens narrows. The posteriorly rotated lateral mass assumes a truncated configuration. See also Figures 8.2, 8.3, 8.6, 8.7, and 8.8.

CHAPTER 3

CLASSIFICATION OF ACUTE CERVICAL SPINE INJURIES

Classification of acute injuries involving the cervical spine and based upon the mechanism of injury or the appearance of the cervical spine in the lateral radiograph have been described or suggested by Holdsworth (19), Beatson (20), Whitley and Forsyth (21), Apley (22), and Babcock (23). These classifications have not proven entirely satisfactory in the everyday management of acute cervical spine injuries because of being (a) too complex, (b) over-simplified, or (c) exclusive of some cervical injuries.

In addition, and unfortunately, some authors have classified the "burst" fracture and the flexion tear-drop fracture as the same lesion. Cheshire (24) has noted that both Beatson (20) and Holdsworth (25) have designated illustrations of flexion tear-drop fractures as burst fractures. This imprecision is repeated by Bedbrook (26) who, in describing "compression" (burst) fractures, states, "these injuries, sometimes known as 'tear-drop' fractures in the cervical spine, are always stable . . . ". More recently, Rothman and Simeone (27) have indicated that "burst fractures, vertical compression fractures, and tear-drop fractures are, for practical purposes, synonymous."

The distinction between the compression (burst) fracture and the flexion tear-drop fracture may be difficult, radiographically. If the degree of flexion is insufficient to produce the classic roentgen appearance of the tear-drop fracture, it may resemble the burst fracture in the lateral view. However, the instability of the flexion tear-drop fracture and its resultant common association of significant neurologic complications should help distinguish the lesions, clinically. Cheshire (24) suggests that the demonstration of instability on lateral flexion and extension radiographs made following conservative therapy establishes the true nature of the lesion. With this exception, most authors agree that the typical burst and flexion tear-drop fractures are sufficiently radiographically characteristic to provide definitive identification. Also, most agree that the distinction is clinically important (21,22,28–32).

For these reasons, it seems appropriate to propose the following classification of acute cervical spine injuries based upon the mechanism of injury. The classification has been formulated on the pragmatic notion that each of the types of injury is caused by a pure, or dominant, mechanism of injury (flexion, extension, vertical compression) or a combination of pure forces (flexion-rotation and extension-rotation). This classification has proven to be simple, practical, and inclusive (Table I).

In addition to recognizing and identifying the type of acute cervical spine injury, it is equally as important to be aware of the stability, or lack of stability, of the lesion. The practical significance of this observation is to have an awareness of those lesions which are frequently

TABLE I
Cervical Spine Injuries: Mechanism of Injury

A. Flexion
   1. Anterior subluxation
   2. Bilateral interfacetal dislocation
   3. Simple wedge fracture
   4. Clay-shoveler's fracture
   5. Flexion tear-drop fracture
B. Flexion-rotation
   1. Unilateral interfacetal dislocation
C. Extension-rotation
   1. Pillar fracture
D. Vertical compression
   1. Bursting fracture
     (a) Jefferson fracture of atlas
     (b) Burst fracture, lower cervical vertebrae
E. Extension
   1. Extension tear-drop fracture
   2. Posterior neural arch fracture, atlas
   3. Hangman's fracture (deceleration, hyperextension)
   4. Hyperextension fracture-dislocation

associated with neurologic damage at the time of injury and to be cognizant of those fractures and dislocations in which unguarded patient motion is liable to produce or aggravate spinal cord or nerve root injury. Therefore, it is basic to the interpretation of the roentgen examination of the acutely injured cervical spine to be aware of those characteristics of the injury which result in loss of stability.

As with other aspects of cervical spine injury, there is not complete accord concerning the definition of stability (or instability), the extent of the injury or the components involved in the injury that affect stability, or even those lesions which are stable and those which are not. Stability is sometimes used in reference to the acute lesion when first seen, sometimes to the acute lesion following initial treatment, and sometimes to the status of the lesion following conservative therapy, "late instability" (24). Stability (or lack of stability) in the current context shall refer to the status of the acute lesion as recorded on the initial roentgen examination.

Stability, with reference to the cervical spine, means that the integrity of the ligamento-skeletal components of the cervical spine has been sufficiently maintained, following trauma, that further controlled motion has a low degree of probability of producing, or aggravating existing cord or nerve root damage. Conversely, Fielding and Hawkins (33) have defined *instability* as "weakness of intervertebral bonds that renders them unable to withstand trauma tolerable to the normal spine and allows actual or potential abnormal excursion of one segment on another, implying potential or actual compromise of neural elements." Apley (22) states, simply, "In stable fractures the cord is rarely damaged and movement of the spine is safe. In unstable fractures, the cord may have been damaged but, if it has escaped, it may be injured by subsequent movement."

While it must be recognized that stability cannot be predicted in every instance of acute cervical injury, there is a practical reason to make as informed an estimation of stability as possible. To do otherwise would require considering all acute cervical injuries as either stable or unstable, neither of which is appropriate. A classification of acute cervical spine injuries, based upon their stability, or lack of stability, is contained in Table II.

Holdsworth (19), Beatson (20), Apley (22), and the majority of other authors relate stability to the integrity of the posterior ligamentous complex, maintaining that if that complex is intact, or only partially disrupted, the lesion is stable. This tenet may be modified if the injury disrupts the intervertebral disk, the anterior longitudinal ligament, the facets bilaterally at the same level, or the bony neural ring. Bedbrook

TABLE II
Cervical Spine Injuries: Degree of Stability

A. Stable
  1. Anterior subluxation
  2. Unilateral interfacetal dislocation
  3. Simple wedge fracture
  4. Burst fracture, lower cervical vertebrae
  5. Posterior neural arch fracture, atlas
  6. Pillar fracture
  7. Clay-shoveler's fracture
B. Unstable
  1. Bilateral interfacetal dislocation
  2. Flexion tear-drop fracture
  3. Extension tear-drop fracture (stable in flexion, unstable in extension)
  4. Hangman's fracture
  5. Jefferson fracture of atlas
  6. Hyperextension fracture-dislocation

(26), on the other hand, contends that the posterior ligament complex is relatively unimportant in this regard and that it is not until the intervertebral disk is completely divided and the anterior longitudinal ligament stripped that the vertebral column becomes "potentially unstable."

"Late instability" has relevance to the current discussion only through its unique incidence in anterior subluxation of the cervical spine. Cheshire (24) has reported an incidence of late instability of 21% in relation to anterior subluxation as compared to an incidence of 5–7% in all other types of cervical injuries. This magnitude of delayed complication underscores the importance of accepting the entity of subluxation and of recognizing its roentgen features.

CHAPTER 4

FLEXION INJURIES

The mechanism of these injuries is presumed to be pure, acute flexion. Selecki (34) has demonstrated, experimentally, that the extent, or type, of flexion injury is directly related to the magnitude of the causative force and to the position and degree of flexion of the spine. The same research has established that the most extensive destruction occurs following direct injury when the head and neck are in the flexed position and that such injuries are characteristic and consist of "drop" or "tear" fractures. Less extensive damage occurs when the spine is in a more neutral attitude and is driven into flexion by the force of injury.

A. ANTERIOR SUBLUXATION

Although Whitley and Forsyth (21) have described some of the roentgen signs of subluxation ("partial dislocation"), anterior subluxation of the cervical spine is a diagnosis commonly held in disrespect, if not frankly rejected, by most radiologists. However, the lesion is obviously recognized by orthopedists and neurosurgeons (34–38). Stringa (39), Holdsworth (19), and Selecki (34) have described the mechanism and pathophysiology of the lesion. Braakman and Penning (40), referring to anterior subluxation as "hyperflexion sprain," have prepared a classic and detailed description of the lesion. Cheshire (24) reported 21% delayed instability following anterior subluxation compared with from 5–7% associated with all other types of cervical injuries. Jackson (38) cites the development of localized degenerative changes following anterior subluxation as evidence of soft tissue trauma at the time of injury.

Anterior subluxation is the result of the least amount of flexion force capable of producing radiographically recognizable cervical spine injury. This lesion consists solely of disruption of the posterior ligament complex (the supra- and interspinous ligaments, the interfacetal joint capsules, and the posterior longitudinal ligament) (Fig. 4.1) (19, 34). Fibers of the posterior portion of the intervertebral disk are only partially disrupted while the anterior longitudinal ligament remains intact. This posteriorly localized, soft tissue damage allows the vertebra immediately above the level of the soft tissue injury to [1] rotate anteriorly, pivoting on its anterior inferior corner or [2] glide anteriorly with respect to the vertebra immediately subjacent to the level of injury.

Because the anterior longitudinal ligament remains intact and because the intervertebral disk is not completely disrupted, anterior subluxation is stable at the time of injury.

The roentgen diagnosis of anterior subluxation, particularly where the involved vertebra is not frankly anteriorly displaced, may be very difficult because of the subtlety of the radiographic findings and because some of the characteristics of anterior subluxation may be simulated by straightening the normal cervical lordotic curve voluntarily (the "military" position) or involuntarily (muscle spasm). Careful evaluation of the lateral radiograph in neutral, flexion, and extension positions, and strict adherence to the criteria of anterior subluxation are necessary to minimize "over-reading." For example, Figure 4.2 depicts the roentgen appearance of the cervical spine of a 16-year-old girl who was involved in an automobile accident in which the car in which she was a passenger was struck from behind. She complained of diffuse pain in the cervical area and moderate limitation of motion. There were no localized signs

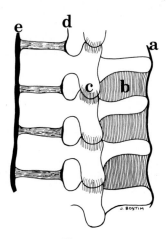

Figure 4.1
Schematic representation of the posterior ligament complex. (a) represents the supraspinous ligament, (b) the interspinous ligament, (c) the capsule of the facetal joint, (d) the posterior longitudinal ligament, and (e) the anterior longitudinal ligament.

or symptoms. In the neutral lateral radiograph (Fig. 4.2a) the normal cervical lordotic curve is reversed uniformly throughout the length of the cervical spine. The interspinous spaces are of similar width and the relationship of the articular facets, and their contiguous posterior cortical margins, are normal and uniform. To the degree that flexion and extension were possible, movement of the vertebral bodies, and their posterior elements, with respect to each other, is physiologic (Fig. 4.2, b and c). Thus, although this patient sustained a flexion-type injury of

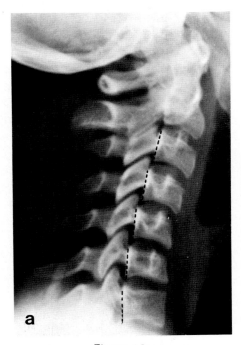

Figure 4.2
Lateral radiographs of the cervical spine made in (a) neutral, (b) flexion, and (c) extension. This patient developed severe pain and limitation of motion of the neck following a rear-ended auto accident. The neutral lateral radiograph (a) demonstrates only smooth, diffuse reversal of the normal cervical lordotic curve. The interspinous spaces from C_3–C_7 are uniformly widened, the anatomy of the interfacetal joints is normal at each level, and each succeedingly higher vertebra has moved forward a slightly greater distance than the subjacent segment resulting in the diffusely reversed curve. All of these findings are the result of muscle spasm. Lateral flexion (b) and extension (c) views record only the physiologic attitude of the cervical spine in those positions. The purpose of this illustration is to emphasize that even when the mechanism of injury and the clinical findings suggest anterior subluxation, the diagnosis rests not upon simple reversal of the normal cervical lordosis, but upon strict adherence to the radiographic criteria of anterior subluxation. This illustration should be compared to Figures 4.3, 4.6, 4.7, 4.8, and 4.9.

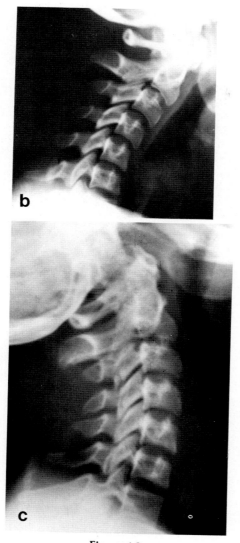

Figure 4.2

the cervical spine, had pain and limitation of motion and, in the neutral lateral radiograph, had *generalized* reversal of the cervical lordotic curve, none of the criteria of subluxation were present, even when the spine was "stressed" by flexion and extension. Therefore, although this patient may have experienced a soft tissue injury in the cervical region, there is no radiographic evidence of anterior subluxation.

Further, the clinical condition of the patient is important in the evaluation of the radiographs. Patients with acute subluxation have

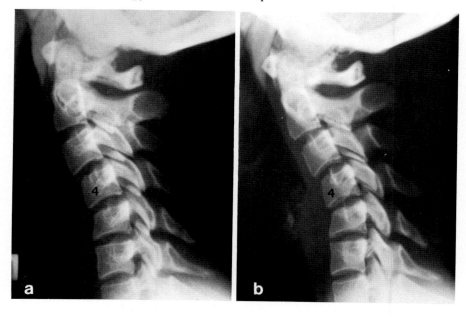

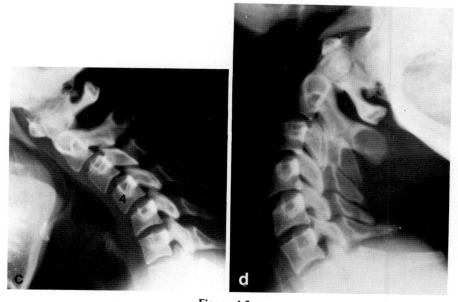

Figure 4.3
(a) Anterior subluxation of C_4 on C_5 sustained at the time of initial injury. (b) Lateral neutral radiograph of the same patient several months later following minor trauma to the neck. The anterior subluxation persists. Flexion (c) and extension (d) views demonstrate delayed instability.

severe pain and marked limitation of flexion and extension. Delayed instability of previous subluxation is relatively pain-free and is not characterized by marked limitation of motion. This concept is illustrated by the history of a patient who sustained an acute anterior subluxation of C$_{4-5}$ which was associated with severe pain and marked limitation of motion, as the result of an automobile accident. Several months later, the patient fell, striking her head and neck on soft ground. She had minimal discomfort and no limitation of motion. The roentgen examination demonstrated the original anterior subluxation and its persistent deformity and instability (Fig. 4.3).

The pathology of anterior subluxation is schematically represented in Figures 4.4 and 4.5. Figure 4.4 represents subluxation in which the involved vertebra simply rotates anteriorly, pivoting on its antero-inferior corner. Figure 4.5 represents the concept of subluxation described by Holdsworth (19) in which there is frank anterior displacement of the vertebral body and disruption, *but not dislocation,* of the interfacetal joints.

Radiographically, the cardinal feature of anterior subluxation which distinguishes it from the physiologic attitude of the cervical spine in the

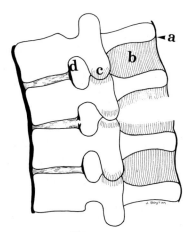

Figure 4.4

Schematic representation of the pathology of subluxation without forward displacement of the subluxed vertebra. The posterior ligament complex (supraspinous ligament [a], interspinous ligament [b], facetal joint ca$_r$sule [c], a:.d posterior longitudinal ligament [d]) is disrupted and there is a short tear into the intervertebral disk. The antero-inferior corner of the vertebral body acts as the pivotal point for the anterior rotation of the involved segment which results in the superior facet of the involved apophyseal joint gliding superiorly and anteriorly with respect to its contiguous inferior facet. (Reprinted by permission from Harris, J. H. Jr.: Acute injuries of the spine. *Semin. Roentgenol.* 13:53, 1978.)

straight (military) or flexion position is the fact that the alteration in alignment of the cervical segments is abrupt and limited to the level of the soft tissue injury. Physiologic changes in alignment of the cervical vertebrae associated with position, or muscle spasm, are distributed in a normal, predictable fashion throughout the length of the cervical spine. This concept is illustrated by comparing the alignment of the cervical vertebrae in Figures 1.17 (normal lateral), 1.24 (normal flexion), 4.2a (muscle spasm), and 4.7a and 4.8a (anterior subluxation).

> *In the following discussion, the term "superior facet" refers to the superior facet of the interfacetal (apophyseal) joint, i.e., the inferior facet of the vertebra above, and "inferior facet" (of the joint) refers to the superior facet of the vertebra below.*

At the level of subluxation, the interspinous space is abnormally wide as the result of disruption of the supraspinous and interspinous ligaments. Increase in width of the interspinous space has been called "fanning" (33). The superior facets of the apophyseal joint are displaced

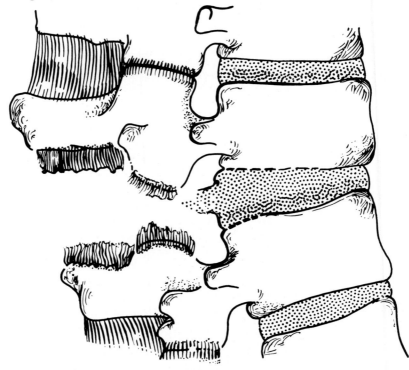

Figure 4.5
Schematic representation of the pathology of anterior subluxation as depicted by Holdsworth (8).

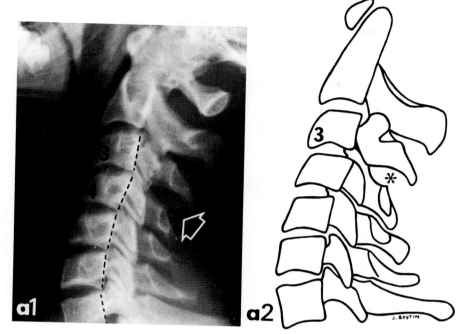

Figure 4.6

Subtle anterior subluxation of C_3 on C_4 in a high school wrestler who sustained a flexion injury. In the neutral lateral projection (a), the sweep of the cervical lordosis is interrupted at the C_{3-4} level, the interspinous space is widened (open arrow), and the intervertebral disk space is narowed anteriorly. In flexion (b), C_3 is clearly anteriorly displaced causing the third interspace to become narrower anteriorly and wider posteriorly while the superior facets of the apophyseal joints at this level glide upward and forward on the inferior facets (small open arrow), and the interspinous space demonstrates greater fanning. In extension (c), all of the signs described in the neutral and flexion positions are reduced and the spine appears normal. (Reprinted by permission from Harris, J. H. Jr. & Harris, W. H.: *The Radiology of Emergency Medicine.* Williams & Wilkins, Baltimore, Md., © 1975.)

upward and forward with respect to their contiguous inferior facets. This movement of the superior facets is evidenced by the increased distance between the posterior cortical margins of the facets at the level of subluxation in comparison to that at the uninvolved levels. Although the superior facets are displaced they remain in their normal posterior position relative to the inferior facets of the apophyseal joint.

The intervertebral disk space becomes widened posteriorly and narrowed anteriorly as a result of forward rotation of the involved vertebral body.

The sum of these changes indicates an injury to soft tissues resulting

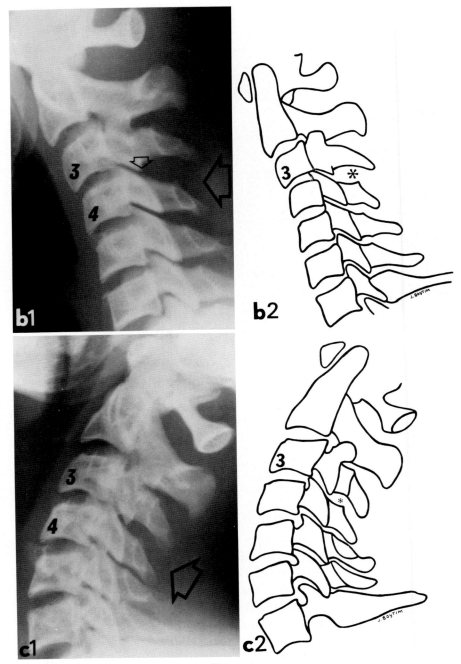

Figure 4.6

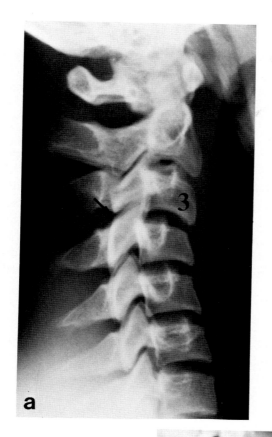

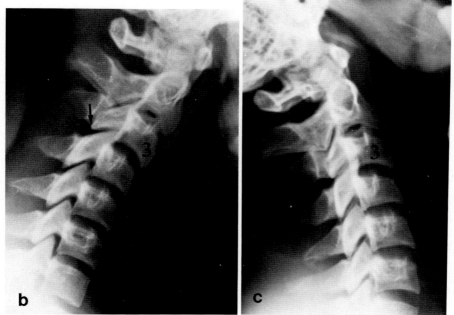

Figure 4.7

in disruption of the normal cervical lordotic curve which is localized to the level of injury.

The involved vertebral body may, or may not, be displaced anteriorly with respect to the subjacent vertebra.

All of the roentgen signs of anterior subluxation are accentuated in flexion and reduced in extension.

Figures 4.6, 4.7, and 4.8 illustrate various degrees of anterior subluxation.

The roentgen evidence of the effects of delayed instability are seen in Figure 4.9. The morbidity of delayed instability following subluxation is sufficient to warrant emphasizing, by repetition, Cheshire's observations that: (a) delayed instability occurs more commonly as a complication of subluxation than any other type of cervical spine injury; and (b) the incidence of delayed instability following subluxation is approximately 21% (24).

B. BILATERAL INTERFACETAL DISLOCATION

The majority of authors believe that bilateral interfacetal dislocation (BID) is the result of a hyperflexion injury (21, 28, 32, 33, 40, 41). Others (19, 24, 29, 42) contend that BID results from combined flexion and rotational forces. All authors agree that both unilateral and bilateral interfacetal dislocations are primarily soft tissue injuries involving principally the posterior ligament complex. Since the roentgen appearance of bilateral interfacetal dislocation contains no intimation of a rotational component, since the bilateral dislocation is reduced by straight traction, and since bilateral interfacetal dislocation has been experimentally produced by a flexion mechanism, it seems appropriate to consider bilateral interfacetal dislocation as a flexion injury.

Bilateral interfacetal dislocation is the result of complete disruption of the posterior ligament complex, including the posterior longitudinal ligament, the annulus, and frequently the anterior longitudinal ligament (20), and anterior dislocation of the superior facets of the interfacetal

---

Figure 4.7
Anterior subluxation of C_3 on C_4. In the neutral (a) and flexion (b) lateral projections, the roentgen signs of anterior subluxation are clearly evident. These include anterior displacement of the body of C_3, anterior narrowing and posterior widening of the disk space, forward displacement of the superior facets of the apophyseal joints (arrow) and fanning (*). The changes in relationship of the facets of the apophyseal joints are well demonstrated, particularly when compared with the facetal joints at the lower levels. In extension (c), all of the signs of anterior subluxation are reversed and the spine appears normal.

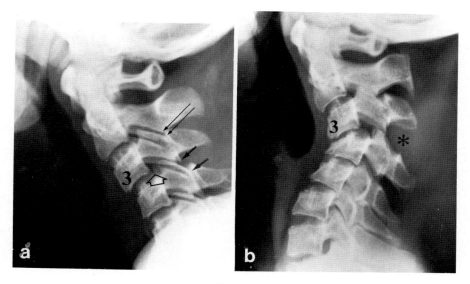

Figure 4.8
Anterior subluxation of C_3 on C_4. In the neutral lateral radiograph made at the time of acute injury (a), the forward displacement of C_3 is obvious. Since the entire vertebra is anteriorly subluxed, the space between the posterior cortex of the body of C_3 and the anterior cortex of the articular masses of C_4 has increased (open arrow) and the superior facet of the involved apophyseal joint has moved forward on its inferior facet. The short-stemmed arrows indicate the distance between the posterior margins of the articular facets of one apophyseal joint at the level of subluxation. The long-stemmed arrows indicate this distance at a normal apophyseal joint. (b) The neutral lateral radiograph of the same patient 8 months later recorded one complication of anterior subluxation. (Reprinted by permission from Harris, J. H. Jr.: Acute injuries of the spine. *Semin. Roentgenol.* 13:53, 1978.)

joint with respect to the inferior facets at the level of injury. The dislocated facets pass upward, forward, and over the inferior facets of the joint and come to rest in the intervertebral foramina.

Bilateral interfacetal dislocation may be partial (incomplete) or complete. When the dislocation is incomplete, the dislocated vertebra will be anteriorly displaced a distance less than one-half the antero-posterior diameter of the vertebral body and the superior facets of the joint, although dislocated anterior to their contiguous inferior facets, sit high in the intervertebral foramina (Fig. 4.10a). Oblique radiographs establish the bilaterality of the dislocation (Fig. 4.10, b and c).

Beatson (20) has demonstrated experimentally that complete bilateral interfacetal dislocation can occur only with total disruption of the posterior ligament complex, the disk, and the anterior longitudinal ligament, and that under these conditions, the dislocated vertebral body

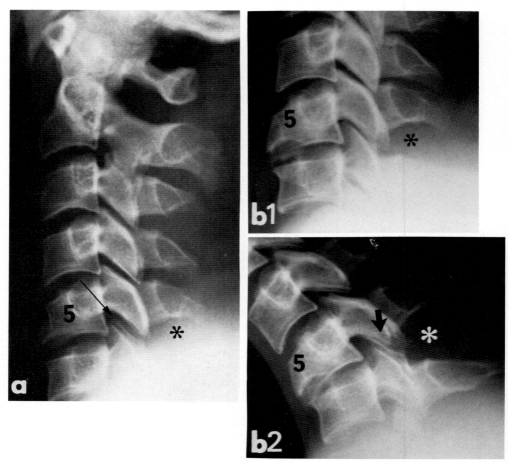

Figure 4.9
Anterior subluxation of C_5 on C_6 associated with a wedge fracture of C_5. While the wedge fracture is the most striking abnormality, the signs of anterior subluxation are evident (a). The fifth vertebra is slightly anteriorly displaced and rotated on its inferior corner, the C_{5-6} disk space is widened (arrow) and, even though incompletely visualized, the interspinous space appears widened (*). Lateral neutral (b1) and flexion (b2) views made 18 months following the original injury indicate the delayed instability at this level by the abnormal forward displacement of C_5 in flexion (b2). The interspinous space is widened (*), the inferior facets of C_5 are displaced forward (arrow), and the disk space is widened posteriorly and narrowed anteriorly.

is anteriorly displaced a distance greater than one-half the antero-posterior diameter of the vertebral body. Beatson's cadaver experiments have established that it is impossible for bilateral interfacetal dislocation to exist without this degree of displacement of the vertebral body and,

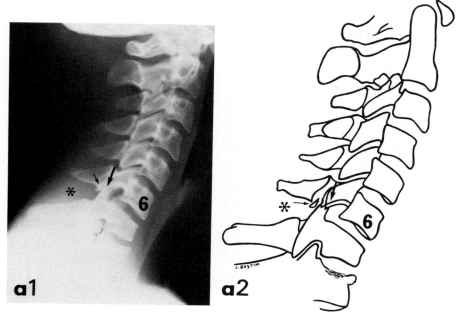

Figure 4.10
Incomplete bilateral interfacetal dislocation. In the lateral radiograph (a), the dislocated sixth segment is anteriorly displaced. The superior facet of each apophyseal joint (large arrow) lies anterior to its contiguous inferior facet. A tiny fracture fragment remains posterior to the inferior facet (small arrow). The interspinous space is abnormally wide (*). Incidental wedge fractures involve the bodies of C_7 and T_1. The oblique projections (b and c) confirm that on each side, the dislocated superior facet of the joint lies within the intervertebral foramen anterior to its corresponding inferior facet. (Reprinted by permission from Harris, J. H. Jr.: Acute injuries of the spine. *Semin. Roentgenol.* 13:53, 1978.)

consequently, that when this degree of anterior displacement of the vertebral body is seen in the lateral radiograph, it is characteristic of bilateral interfacetal dislocation.

Frequently, a small fracture, generally involving one of the facets, can be demonstrated radiographically. Bedbrook (26) verified the presence of a fracture in each of the 70 patients with cervical spine dislocation examined at autopsy or surgical exploration. The fracture was commonly not visible radiographically. In view of the extensive soft tissue injury associated with BID, these fractures are of little clinical significance.

Bilateral interfacetal dislocation, because of its extensive soft tissue damage and dislocated facetal joints, is unstable and is associated with a high incidence of cord damage (20, 22, 35, 41).

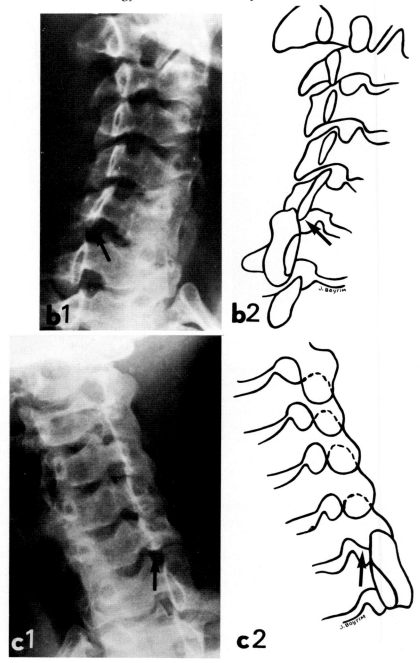

Figure 4.10

C. Wedge Fracture

More forceful flexion trauma results in the simple wedge fracture of a vertebral body (34), generally in the mid or lower cervical segments. The posterior ligament complex is stretched, but remains intact. The intervertebral disk and the anterior longitudinal ligament are intact. The integrity of the interfacetal joints is maintained. Wedge fracture, therefore, is a stable lesion.

The wedge fracture is caused by mechanical compression of the involved vertebra between the adjacent vertebral bodies. In the lateral radiograph, the lesion is characterized by a loss of stature of the involved vertebra anteriorly and by an increase in the width of the prevertebral soft tissues, reflecting the presence of hemorrhage (Fig. 4.11a). In the antero-posterior projection, the involved vertebra may be of normal or decreased stature (Fig. 4.11b). The absence of a vertical fracture line in the vertebral body with a wedge fracture helps distinguish the wedge fracture from the burst fracture.

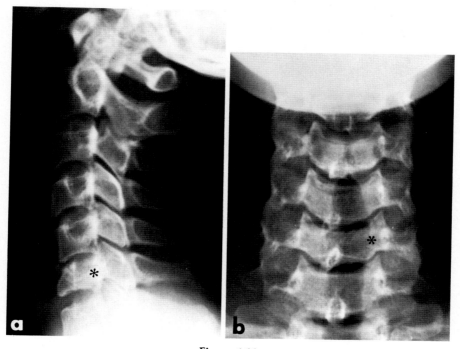

Figure 4.11
Wedge fracture of C_6 (*). In the lateral projection (a), the anterior portion of the body is decreased in stature while posteriorly the height is normal. In the frontal projection (b), the vertebral body is decreased in stature, but does not contain a vertical fracture line.

D. CLAY-SHOVELER'S FRACTURE

The clay-shoveler's fracture, also called "coal miner's" fracture, "shoveler's disease," or "shoveler's" fracture, is an avulsion-type of injury which involves the spinous process of C₇, C₆, or T₁, in that order of frequency. This injury is the result of an abrupt flexion of the head and neck against the tense "set" of the posterior ligaments causing an oblique fracture of the proximal portion of the spinous process (Fig. 4.12). The clay-shoveler's fracture is stable.

E. FLEXION TEAR-DROP FRACTURE-DISLOCATION

The most severe flexion force produces the "flexion tear-drop fracture," which is the most severe injury of the cervical spine compatible with life. This lesion, described by Schneider and Kahn in 1956 (31) derives its name from the characteristic triangle-shaped separate frag-

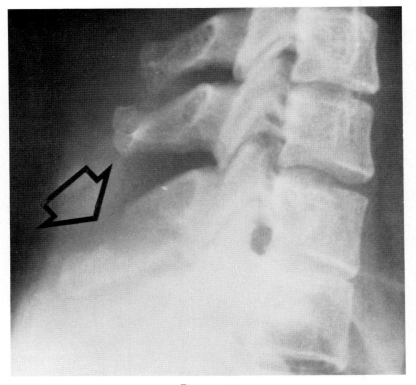

Figure 4.12
Clay-shoveler's fracture. (Reprinted by permission from Harris, J. H. Jr. & Harris, W. H.: *The Radiology of Emergency Medicine.* Williams & Wilkins, Baltimore, Md. © 1975; and Harris, J. H. Jr.: Acute injuries of the spine. *Semin. Roentgenol.* 13:53, 1978.)

ment that arises from the anterior-inferior corner of the vertebral body. This fragment has been likened to a tear falling from a cheek.

Clinically, the flexion tear-drop fracture is frequently associated with the "acute anterior cervical cord syndrome" (43, 44) which consists of immediate complete quadraplegia, loss of pain and temperature sensations (anterior column senses), but with retention of the posterior column senses of position, motion, and vibration.

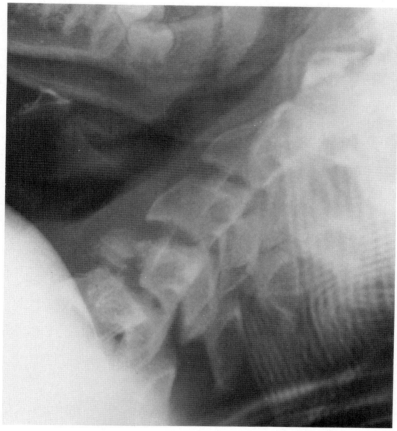

Figure 4.13

Flexion tear-drop fracture of C_4. The spine is flexed above the level of the injury and marked posterior angulation is present at the level of injury. The triangle-shaped anterior fragment is displaced anteriorly resulting in the characteristic tear-drop configuration. The fragmentation and position of the vertebral body indicate that the anterior longitudinal ligament, the intervertebral disk, and the posterior longitudinal ligament are disrupted. Posteriorly, the interfacetal joints are subluxed and the interspinous space is widened indicating disruption of the posterior ligament complex. (Reprinted by permission from Harris, J. H. Jr.: Acute injuries of the spine. *Semin. Roentgenol.* 13:53, 1978.)

Radiographically (Fig. 4.13), the attitude of the spine is that of flexion from the level of the injury upward. The involved vertebral body is fractured with the anterior-inferior corner constituting the "tear-drop" fragment. The spinal canal is narrowed, at the level of injury, by posterior angulation of the cervical column and posterior displacement of the involved vertebral body. Consequently, the spinal canal is severely compromised.

In lateral projection, the involved vertebra is displaced and rotated anteriorly and, depending upon the degree and magnitude of flexion at the instant of injury, the interfacetal joints may be bilaterally subluxed or dislocated. The anterior and posterior longitudinal ligaments, the intervertebral disk, and the posterior ligamentous complex are disrupted. Therefore, the flexion tear-drop fracture is completely unstable.

The correct identification and designation of flexion tear-drop fractures and of burst (compression, dispersion) fractures are of fundamental clinical importance because of the significant difference in neurologic involvement, stability, and management. The flexion tear-drop fracture is caused by severe flexion (45), has a typical radiographic appearance, is completely unstable, and is commonly associated with the acute anterior cervical cord syndrome. The burst fracture, on the other hand, is caused by a vertical compression mechanism of injury directed through the straightened cervical spine, is characterized by comminution of the centrum, is stable and, although a posterior fragment may impinge upon the cord (22), neurologic involvement is generally not a major feature of this fracture.

CHAPTER 5

FLEXION- AND EXTENSION-ROTA-TION INJURIES

A. FLEXION-ROTATION

1. Unilateral Interfacetal Dislocation

Whereas pure, or dominant, flexion force produces a variety of acute cervical spine injuries, including bilateral interfacetal dislocation, the simultaneous flexion-rotation mechanism produces only the unilateral interfacetal dislocation (UID). An interfacetal joint on the side of the direction of rotation acts as the pivotal point while the superior facet of a contralateral apophyseal joint rides upward, forward, and over the tip of the contiguous inferior facet of the involved joint, coming to rest in the intervertebral foramen anterior to the inferior facet of the joint. In this position the dislocated facet is mechanically "locked" (46) in place. The UID is, because of the locked attitude of the dislocated facet, stable, even though the posterior ligament complex, including the capsule of the involved joint, is disrupted and the posterior longitudinal ligament and annulus are partially disrupted. Braakman and Vinken (46) note that the capsule of the nondislocated facetal joint is also disrupted and the inferior facet of the dislocated joint is frequently fractured. Beatson (20) has demonstrated experimentally that it is impossible to produce

61

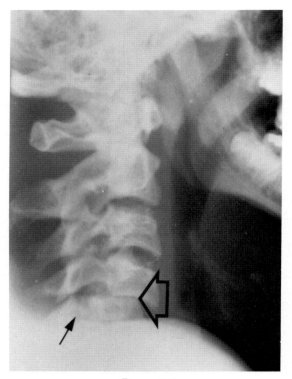

Figure 5.1
Unilateral interfacetal dislocation (UID). The forward displacement of the dislocated vertebra is less than one-half the antero-posterior diameter of the vertebral body (open arrow). The dislocated superior facet of the involved joint (small arrow) is visible in the intervertebral foramen, anterior to its corresponding inferior facet. (Reprinted by permission from Harris, J. H. Jr. & Harris, W. H.: *The Radiology of Emergency Medicine.* Williams & Wilkins, Baltimore, Md., © 1975.)

Figure 5.2
(a_1) UID of C_5 on C_6. The dislocated vertebra is anteriorly displaced a distance less than one-half the antero-posterior diameter of the vertebral body. The posterior inferior corner of the dislocated superior facet (open arrow) is visible anterior to its contiguous inferior facet, seated in the intervertebral foramen. Above the level of dislocation, all of the facetal joints on the side of the dislocation, because of the rotational component of the injury, lie anterior to the contralateral facetal joint. Each set of arrows indicates the location of the facetal joints at the same level. In the schematic representation (a_2), the facetal joints on the side of the dislocation are indicated by the broken line. (b) In the left posterior oblique projection, the dislocated superior facet (arrow) is seen in the intervertebral foramen. (c) In the right posterior oblique projection, the contralateral, nondisplaced lamina (arrow) is slightly superiorly and anteriorly situated with respect to the subjacent lamina, but remains posterior to the subjacent lamina.

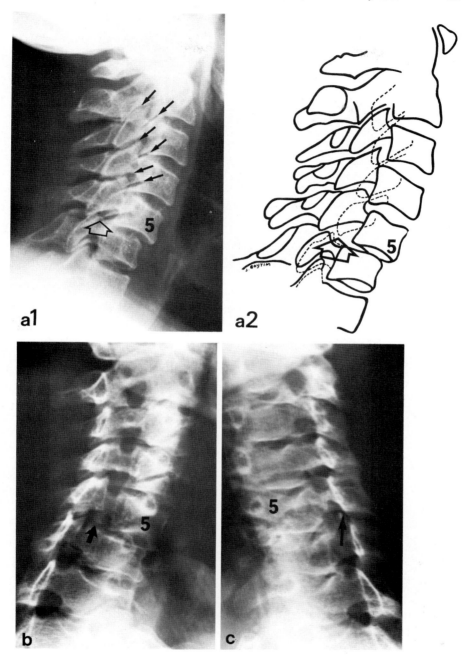

Figure 5.2

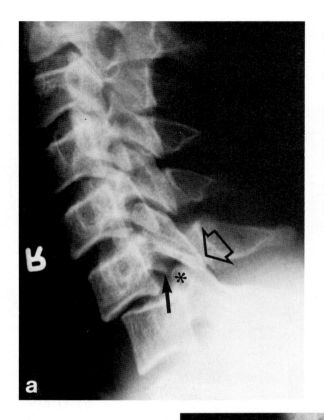

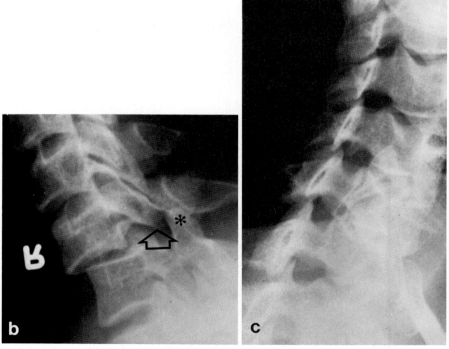

Figure 5.3

forward displacement of the involved vertebra of more than one-half the width of a vertebral body in the presence of a UID.

> *The reader is reminded that "superior facet" refers to the superior facet of the apophyseal joint, i.e., the anatomic inferior facet of the upper vertebra.*

Radiographically, in the neutral lateral projection, the dislocated vertebral body is anteriorly displaced a distance less than one-half the antero-posterior diameter of a vertebral body (Fig. 5.1).

The rotational component of the mechanism of injury is indicated by the fact that the articular pillars and the interfacetal joints, at the level of the dislocation and above, are no longer superimposed. The dislocated articular mass, being rotated anteriorly, is partially superimposed upon, and obscured by, the vertebral body. All of the vertebrae above the level of dislocation are similarly rotated and present an identical roentgen appearance. The posterior inferior margin of the dislocated superior facet may be seen lying in the intervertebral foramen anterior to the superior tip of the contiguous inferior facet (Fig. 5.2). The dislocated superior facet may be fractured (Fig. 5.3).

The superior facet of the contralateral apophyseal joint is displaced upward and forward with respect to its contiguous inferior facet so that the joint surfaces are only in partial apposition. However, in spite of this movement, the superior facet remains posterior to the contiguous inferior facet (Figs. 5.2a$_1$, 5.2a$_2$, 5.2c, 5.3a, 5.3c).

The effect of rotation upon the dislocated segment, and those above, is clearly demonstrated with a dried, disarticulated cervical skeleton. Figure 5.4 is the neutral lateral radiograph of such a specimen in which the contiguous articulating surfaces of one of the facetal joints at the C$_{3-4}$ level have been identified by lead foil. It is an important observation that the joint spaces and the posterior cortical surfaces of the articulating pillars, at each level, are superimposed upon one another.

Following dislocation of the marked joint, lateral and oblique radiographs were made of the specimen. The lateral radiograph (Fig. 5.5)

Figure 5.3

Unilateral interfacetal dislocation with a fracture of the dislocated superior facet. (a) Neutral lateral radiograph. The amputated, dislocated superior facet (small arrow) lies anterior to its contiguous inferior facet (*). The contralateral superior facet (open arrow) has glided upward with respect to its contiguous inferior facet, but retains its normal position posterior to the inferior facet. (b) In the right posterior oblique projection, the fractured, dislocated superior facet (arrow) is clearly seen in the intervertebral foramen anterior to its contiguous inferior facet (*). (c) In the opposite oblique projection, the alignment of the laminae is normal.

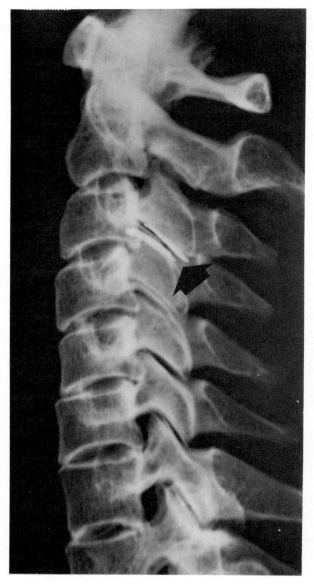

Figure 5.4
Lateral radiograph of dried cervical spine specimen in which the superior and inferior facets of one of the interfacetal joints at the C$_{3-4}$ level have been marked with lead (arrow). The interfacetal joints are superimposed and are situated, normally, posterior to the vertebral body.

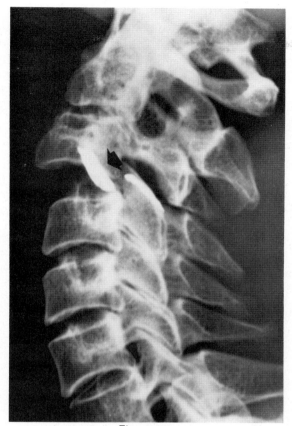

Figure 5.5
 Lateral radiograph following dislocation of the marked facetal joint. The dislocated superior facet (arrow) of the involved joint is clearly anterior to the contiguous inferior facet. Above the level of dislocation, the vertebrae are seen in obliquity. Below the level of the dislocation, the vertebrae are seen in lateral position.

demonstrates that the superior facet of the joint is dislocated anterior to the contiguous inferior facet. Below the level of dislocation, the vertebrae are seen in lateral position. At, and above, the level of dislocation, the vertebrae are seen in oblique position because of the rotational component of the mechanism of injury.

In the oblique radiograph of the same specimen (Fig. 5.6), the dislocated superior facet of the involved joint is clearly evident in the intervertebral foramen anterior to the inferior facet and its articular mass. Due to the effect of rotation, the second and third vertebrae are seen, in this oblique view, in nearly true lateral position.

To illustrate the effect of rotation further, a UID was produced on the same side as the marked joint, but at the next subjacent level, and radiographs were again obtained in lateral and oblique projections.

In the lateral radiograph (Fig. 5.7), the marked facetal joint has been rotated anteriorly, along with all of the vertebrae above the level of the dislocation, and it is superimposed upon the vertebral bodies. Below the level of dislocation, the vertebrae are seen in lateral position, while those above the level of dislocation are recorded in nearly oblique view.

In the oblique projection of this specimen (Fig. 5.8), the vertebrae above the level of the dislocation are seen in lateral projection because of the rotation inherent in this production of UID.

Before proceeding with the discussion of the roentgen findings of UID in the other projections, it is appropriate to re-emphasize the critical importance of the true lateral radiograph of the cervical spine,

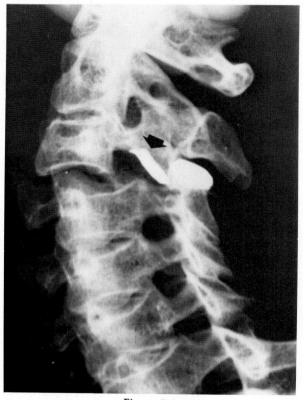

Figure 5.6

Oblique radiograph of same specimen as Figure 5.5. The dislocated superior facet of the involved joint (arrow) lies in the intervertebral foramen. Below the level of the dislocation, the vertebrae are seen in oblique projection. Above the dislocation, the vertebrae are nearly lateral in position.

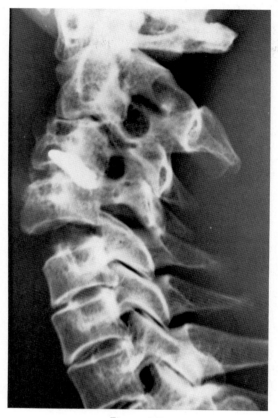

Figure 5.7

Lateral radiograph of dried specimen following unilateral dislocation on the same side as the marked facetal joint, but at the next lower level. Below the dislocation, the vertebrae are seen in lateral projection. Above the dislocation, the rotational component is indicated by the anterior location of the marked facetal joint and by the fact that the upper vertebrae are seen in oblique projection.

the effect of positional rotation upon the lateral radiograph, and its significance in the recognition of UID. This relationship has been described in Chapter 1.

Oblique projections are required in UID in order to identify the side of the dislocation and to evaluate the articular masses and their facets for the presence of associated fracture. Identification of the side of the dislocation is essential to reduction of the lesion.

In the antero-posterior radiograph, the spinous processes above the level of the dislocation are deviated from the midline in the direction of the rotation, *i.e.,* the spinous processes point to the side of the interfacetal dislocation.

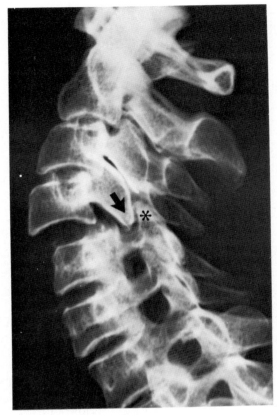

Figure 5.8

Oblique radiograph of the same specimen as Figure 5.7. Below the level of dislocation, the vertebrae are in oblique position. The relationship of the dislocated articular mass (arrow) to the subjacent mass (*) is clear. Above the level of dislocation, because of the rotational component, the vertebrae are seen in true lateral projection.

B. EXTENSION-ROTATION

Combined extension and rotation of the cervical spine has been called "unilateral extension" by Whitley and Forsyth (21). With this mechanism of injury, the maximum force is concentrated upon the apophyseal joints of the mid and lower cervical segments, resulting in a vertical fracture of one of the lateral masses, *i.e.,* the pillar fracture (15, 18, 21). Following the initial impact, it is postulated that the fractures are distracted by rebound flexion of the head and neck.

The pillar fracture is not a common lesion, but Smith (47) believes that the lesion may occur more commonly than has been reported.

Radiographically, the pillar fracture may be easily overlooked on routine frontal and lateral projections. However, subtle findings in each of these views should create the suspicion of a pillar fracture and prompt oblique and pillar views.

In the antero-posterior radiograph (Fig. 5.9), displacement of the pillar fragments can be expected to produce disruption in the smoothly undulating, continuous density of the lateral cortical margins of the superimposed articular masses. The interfacetal joints, not normally visible in the frontal projection, may be partially evident at the level of the fracture (47). The associated soft tissue hematoma may displace the tracheal air shadow on the side of the fracture.

In the lateral roentgenogram, asymmetry of the posterior cortical margins of the articular masses at a single level only indicates posterior displacement of the separate fragment ("double outline" sign [47]). A

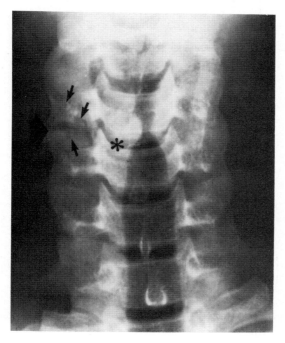

Figure 5.9
Pillar fracture involving the right articular mass of C$_4$. In the frontal projection, the smooth, undulating cortical density caused by the lateral margins of the superimposed articular masses is disrupted and the apophyseal joint is inappropriately visible in this view (arrow). Subtle fracture lines are present (small arrows). The proximal portion of the tracheal air column and its subglottic shoulder is asymmetrical on the right because of the associated hematoma (*).

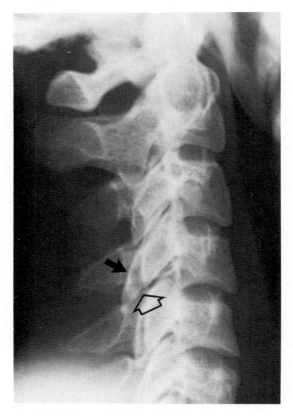

Figure 5.10
In the lateral radiograph, the posterior cortical margins of the articular masses are asymmetrical as a result of the posterior displacement of the separate fragment of the pillar fracture (double outline sign) (arrow). A fracture defect is present in the inferior articulating facet (open arrow).

fracture line, or defect, may be visible in the inferior articulating facet of the involved mass (Fig. 5.10).

The pillar fracture is usually visible in the appropriate oblique projection (Fig. 5.11). However, it may not be apparent in oblique projection if the fragments are neither displaced nor depressed or if the vertical plane of the fracture line does not coincide with the obliquity of the projection.

The pillar view, because it is designed to depict the lateral mass *en face,* is required to evaluate the presence of an articular mass fracture completely and adequately. The fracture typically extends vertically through the articular mass and the separate fragment, or fragments, may be depressed or displaced laterally (Fig. 5.12). Tomography, either in the appropriate oblique position or with the patient supine and the head

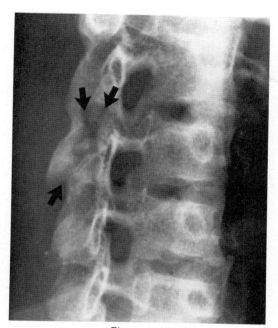

Figure 5.11
Left posterior oblique projection demonstrating the comminuted fracture of the articular mass (arrows).

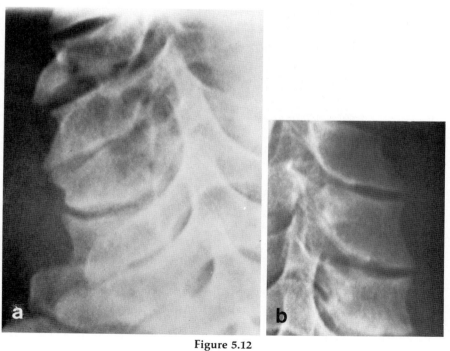

Figure 5.12
Pillar view. The fracture is well seen on the right (a). Note the variation of the height and configuration of the lateral masses on the uninjured, asymptomatic left side (b).

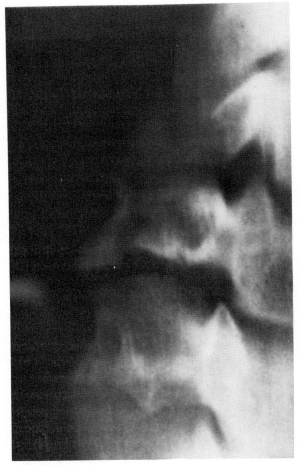

Figure 5.13
The tomogram made with the patient supine and the head turned to the left demonstrates the degree of comminution and the position of the fragments of the pillar fracture.

turned as far as possible toward the uninjured side (Fig. 5.13), enhances demonstration of the pillar fracture.

The diagnosis of an acute pillar fracture requires the demonstration of an acute fracture involving the articular mass. Unilateral compression of an articular mass and asymmetry of lateral masses, in the pillar view, are common radiographic findings, unrelated to patient age and of protean etiology, including developmental. Thus, variations from the normal configuration of the articular mass, alone, and without a demonstrable fracture line, should not be used as evidence of an acute pillar fracture (18, 20).

CHAPTER 6

VERTICAL COMPRESSION INJURIES

Vertical compression injuries are recognized as a distinct type of cervical spine trauma by the great majority of authors. The principal dissention from this consensus is stated by Selecki and Williams (34) who believe that compression is such a major factor in all types of cervical trauma that "any classification of mechanism of injury in which it is implied that there is a single mechanism for compression fractures is bound to confuse the mechanisms with the radiological end results of the injury."

Vertical compression injuries occur only in those segments of the spine that are capable of being voluntarily straightened, *i.e.,* the cervical and lumbar regions (19, 25). Cervical compression injuries are usually the result of force transmitted through the skull and occipital condyles to the spine. They are uncommon because the vertical compression injury must occur at the precise instant that the spine is straight. The same type of force applied through the skull with the spine flexed or extended results in flexion- or extension-type injuries.

Compression injuries of the cervical spine are: (*a*) the Jefferson bursting fracture of the atlas; and (*b*) the "burst" fracture of the lower cervical spine.

A. THE JEFFERSON FRACTURE OF THE ATLAS

The bursting fracture of the atlas was first described by Jefferson (48) in 1920 and as recently as 1970 only 191 cases of this injury had been reported in the world literature (22). The fracture is the result of force transmitted through the occipital condyles to the lateral masses of the atlas. The force drives the articular masses laterally producing bilateral fractures of both the anterior and the posterior arch of C_1 (Fig. 6.1), as well as disruption of the transverse atlantal ligament. The classic Jefferson fracture is characterized by symmetrical bilateral lateral displace-

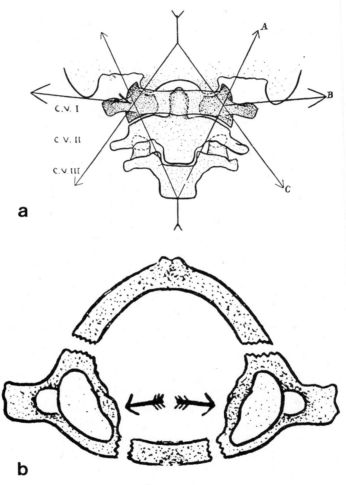

a

b

Figure 6.1
Schematic representation of the forces that produce the Jefferson fracture (a) and of the fracture itself (b). Note that fractures are present bilaterally in both the anterior and the posterior arch. (Reprinted by permission from Jefferson, G.: Fracture of the atlas vertebra. Report of four cases, and a review of those previously recorded. *Br. J. Surg.* 7:407, 1920.)

ment of the articular masses of the atlas. When the causative force is eccentrically applied to the skull and is transmitted in greater magnitude to one lateral mass than the other, the displacement of the articular masses will be asymmetrical (Fig. 6.2).

The Jefferson fracture is commonly associated with acute disruption

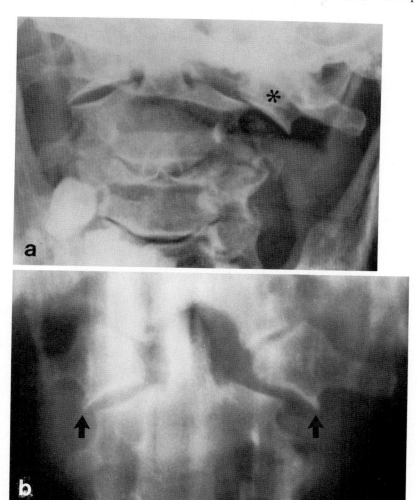

Figure 6.2
Jefferson fracture caused by force eccentrically delivered to the skull resulting in greater displacement of the left lateral mass of the atlas (*) than the right (a). The left lateral mass of the axis is severely comminuted. Lesser fractures involve the left lateral mass of C_2 and C_3, as well. The frontal tomogram (b) confirms the lateral displacement of each articular mass (arrows).

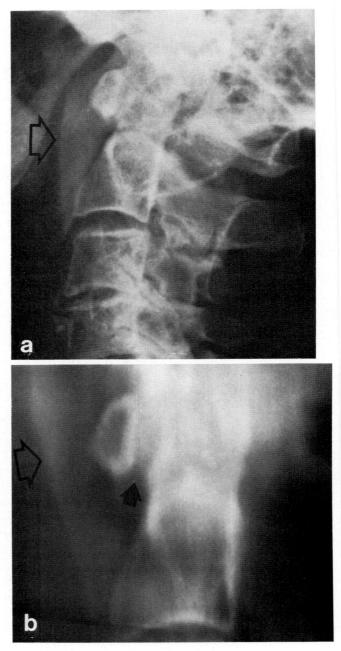

Figure 6.3

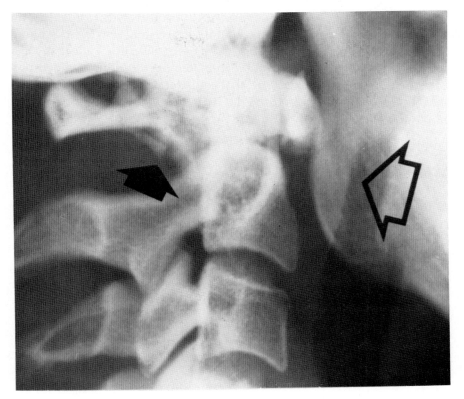

Figure 6.4
Jefferson fracture with minimal displacement of the posterior arch fragments (solid arrow). The most striking roentgen sign of the fracture is the abnormal thickness of the soft tissue shadow anterior to the atlanto-axial articulation (open arrow) caused by the soft tissue hematoma. (Reprinted by permission from Harris, J. H. Jr. & Harris, W. H.: *The Radiology of Emergency Medicine.* Williams & Wilkins, Baltimore, Md., © 1975.)

of the transverse atlantal ligament. Isolated traumatic rupture of the transverse atlantal ligament is rare (11). Transverse atlantal ligament tear is indicated by an atlanto-dental interval (ADI) in excess of 3 mm. Tomograms of the atlanto-axial articulation, made in lateral projection, may be necessary to detect abnormal widening of the ADI (Fig. 6.3).

Figure 6.3
The ADI in this patient with a Jefferson fracture seems normal in the routine lateral radiograph (a). A prevertebral hematoma is present (arrow). The lateral tomogram (b), however, clearly demonstrates abnormal width of the ADI (solid arrow), indicating disruption of the transverse atlantal ligament. The prevertebral soft tissue swelling (open arrow) is evident.

Minimally displaced Jefferson fractures are diffucult to identify on the routine radiographs. In the lateral projection, the most striking roentgen sign may be prevertebral soft tissue swelling caused by the hematoma (Fig. 6.4). In both frontal and lateral projections, tomography is frequently required to establish the bilateral lateral mass displacement, the extent of the fracture (Fig. 6.5), and, as indicated previously, the width of the ADI (Fig. 6.3).

B. "BURST" FRACTURE

The vertical compression injury of the mid or lower cervical segments is referred to as the "burst," "bursting," "compression," or "dispersion" fracture. Roaf (29) has demonstrated, experimentally, that the burst fracture occurs when the nucleus pulposus is imploded into the vertebral body through the inferior end-plate and then explodes the body from

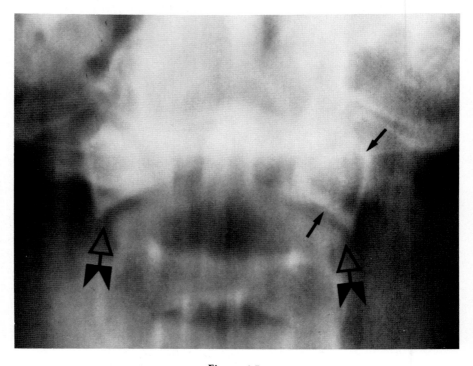

Figure 6.5
The lateral displacement of the lateral masses (winged arrows) of this Jefferson fracture was not apparent on the plain open-mouth view. The small arrows indicate a fracture of the left lateral mass of the atlas which, also, was not visible on the routine radiograph. (Reprinted by permission from Harris, J. H. Jr. & Harris, W. H.: *The Radiology of Emergency Medicine.* Williams & Wilkins, Baltimore, Md., © 1975.)

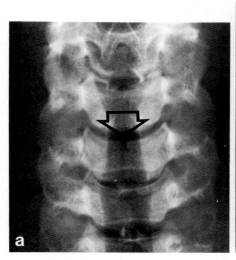 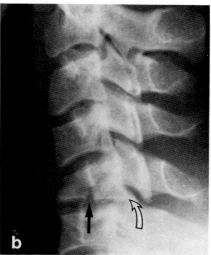

Figure 6.6
"Burst" fracture of C₅ in frontal projection (a). The arrow indicates the vertical
fracture of the vertebral body, which is characteristic of this lesion. In the lateral
projection (b), the cervical vertebrae are in vertical alignment. The body of C₅ is
comminuted with a fracture defect of the inferior end-plate (solid arrow) and posterior
displacement of the posterior body fragment (open arrow). The disk space is narrowed
and the annulus bulges anteriorly. The interfacetal joints at the level of injury are
neither subluxed nor dislocated and the interspinous ligament is intact, as evidenced by
the absence of "fanning" of the interspinous space. Compare this fracture, in lateral
projection, with the flexion tear-drop fracture, Figure 4.13. (Reprinted by permission
from Harris, J. H. Jr. & Harris, W. H.: *The Radiology of Emergency Medicine.* Williams
& Wilkins, Baltimore, Md., © 1975.)

within outward resulting in the characteristic comminuted vertebral
body fracture. Roaf has observed that the annulus of the intervertebral
disk remains intact. The posterior ligament complex remains intact and
the interfacetal joints are normally maintained. Therefore, the burst
fracture is considered stable (19, 22, 25, 26, 41).

Posterior displacement of a posterior or posterior inferior body fragment is characteristic of the burst fracture. This fragment may impinge
upon, or penetrate, the ventral surface of the cord. When the fragment
is small and thin, it may not be visible radiographically (20). While
neurologic signs frequently accompany the burst fracture, the extent,
magnitude, and frequency of cord damage are less than those characteristically associated with the flexion tear-drop fracture.

Radiographically, the burst fracture is characterized, in the frontal
projection, by a vertical fracture line which occurs at the time the

nucleus pulposus is driven through the inferior end-plate (Fig. 6.6a). This feature distinguishes the burst fracture from the wedge fracture which may resemble the burst fracture in the lateral radiograph.

In the lateral radiograph (Fig. 6.6b), the vertebrae are vertically aligned. The fractured vertebral body is comminuted and a posterior fragment typically protrudes into the spinal canal. The interspinous space and the interfacetal joints, at the level of the injury are normal.

CHAPTER 7

EXTENSION INJURIES

The mechanism of extension injuries of the cervical spine is a pure, or dominant, backward force delivered to the spine, usually from a blow or fall on the face or chin. The type of injury depends upon the direction and magnitude of the hyperextensive force.

A. Hyperextension Cervical Injuries with "Normal" Roentgen Examination

Hyperextension dislocation of the cervical spine associated with paraplegia or tetraplegia without roentgen signs of structural damage is a well documented (23, 49) but little appreciated injury which was first recognized by Taylor and Blackwood (50), Taylor (51), and Forsyth (55). The lesion results from a backward and upward force, without a compressive element, delivered to the cervical spine from a blow on the face or forehead. With forced hyperextension, the posterior elements act as a fulcrum. If the hyperextensive force is sufficiently strong, it will cause the anterior longitudinal ligament to rupture. The same force may produce either a tear of the intervertebral disk or separation of the disk from the inferior end-plate of the adjacent superior vertebra. In the latter instance a tiny fracture may be pulled off from the anterior margin of the end-plate.

With continued hyperextension, the vertebrae above the level of the tear in the anterior longitudinal ligament and disk are forced posteriorly and the posterior longitudinal ligament becomes separated from the posterior surface of the subjacent vertebral body. The spinal cord then, becomes compressed between the posteriorly displaced vertebra and the sharp margin of the posterior neural arch formed by the lamina and the invaginated ligamentum flava. The resultant injury to the cervical cord involves, primarily, the posterior column and is characterized by motor loss (52–54).

This type of lesion reduces spontaneously and, typically, the cervical spine is normal in roentgen appearance. Occasionally, a tiny chip fracture arising from the anterior margin of the inferior end-plate of the dislocated vertebra may be visible in the lateral radiograph (50). Hemorrhage associated with the tear of the anterior longitudinal ligament causes diffuse widening of the prevertebral soft tissue shadow (Fig. 7.1) which is the most striking roentgen sign of this injury. A thin lucent shadow ("vacuum defect") may be seen in the anterior aspect of the damaged disk.

The diagnosis of this type of hyperextension injury depends upon a history of the mechanism of injury, the presence of a soft tissue injury of the face or forehead, paraplegia or quadraplegia, and a normal appearing cervical spine. Although the alignment of the cervical vertebrae, including their posterior elements, is normal, diffuse prevertebral soft tissue swelling will be evident. Occasionally, a thin fracture fragment lying within the disk space parallel to the anterior aspect of the inferior end-plate or a "vacuum defect" in the anterior portion of the torn disk may be seen.

The importance of the syndrome of paraplegia with "normal" cervical vertebrae lies in the recognition that it represents a hyperextension injury and that immobilization of the spine in extension may aggravate the existing cervical cord injury.

B. HYPEREXTENSION FRACTURE-DISLOCATION

If the hyperextensive force is combined with a downward (compressive) component, and if the force is eccentrically directed or the head rotated, the resultant injury is the hyperextension fracture-dislocation described by Forsyth (55). In this instance, the force is concentrated on the lateral masses and then to the remainder of the posterior elements on the same side. The articular mass becomes comminuted and fractures may occur in the pedicle and lamina. With continual downward force, the involved vertebra becomes slightly anteriorly displaced. The anterior longitudinal ligament may, or may not, be disrupted.

Radiographically, the undulating seemingly continuous lateral cortical margin of the articular masses is disrupted as a result of the comminuted fracture of the lateral mass. The most important observation is that the involved vertebra is *anteriorly* displaced in the lateral radiograph, even though the mechanism of injury is primarily hyperextension. The

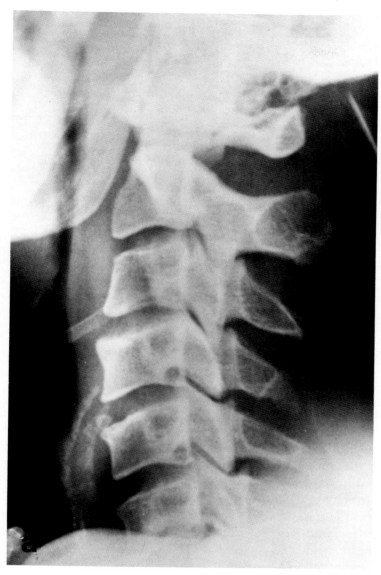

Figure 7.1

(a) Lateral radiograph of the cervical spine of a patient who sustained a hyperextension injury with paresthesias of each extremity. The vertebral bodies and their appendages are intact and of normal alignment. The prevertebral soft tissue shadow, however, is diffusely widened. Cervical myelogram performed shortly post-trauma demonstrates an increase in the transverse diameter of the cord secondary to edema (b). A lateral radiograph made in controlled extension (c), 7 days post-injury, demonstrates anterior widening of the third disk space and a vacuum defect in the anterior portion of the disk (arrow). The prevertebral soft tissue swelling has greatly diminished. (Figure 7.1a and 7.1b appear on page 86.)

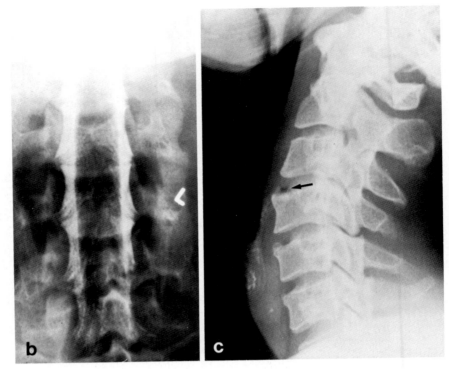

Figure 7.1 B and C

fractured articular mass is characteristically severely comminuted with many small fragments, in contradistinction to the relatively simple pillar fracture. In the appropriate oblique projection, the inferior articulating facet of the fractured articular mass will be seen to be compressed and displaced upward resulting in the "horizontal facet" (55) configuration. Fractures may involve the lamina, pedicle, or spinous process. The tip of the contiguous superior articulating facet of the subjacent vertebra may be fractured (Fig. 7.2). The contralateral interfacetal joint may, or may not, be dislocated.

It is important to be aware that this fracture-dislocation is a hyper-extension injury, even though in the lateral radiograph the anterior displacement of the involved segment suggests a flexion injury, in order that the appropriate management of an extension injury with probable posterior cord damage is instituted.

The hyperextension fracture-dislocation should be considered unsta-ble because of disruption of the posterior elements and the associated ligamentous injury.

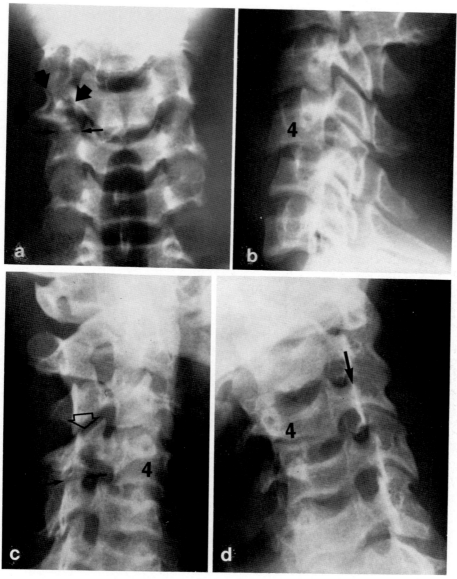

Figure 7.2

Hyperextension fracture-dislocation of C_4. In the frontal projection (a), the severely comminuted fracture of the right lateral mass of C_4 is indicated by the large arrows and the fracture of the superior facet of C_5 by the small arrows. In the lateral radiograph (b), the slight forward displacement of C_4 is evident. The left posterior oblique projection (c) demonstrates the severely comminuted fracture of the right lateral mass of C_4 (open arrow) and the compression and upward displacement of its inferior facetal fragments, producing the "horizontal facet." The small solid arrows indicate the fracture of the superior articulating facet of C_5. The opposite (right posterior) oblique radiograph (d) demonstrates the dislocation of the left interfacetal joint at the C_{4-5} level. The left lamina of C_4 (arrow) is anterior to that of C_5.

C. POSTERIOR ATLANTAL ARCH FRACTURE

Fracture of the posterior arch of the atlas is a relatively common injury that occurs as the result of the posterior arch of C_1 being compressed between the occiput and the heavy posterior arch of the axis during severe hyperextension (56). The fracture involves each side of the posterior arch posterior to the level of the lateral masses and the transverse atlantal ligament. Because the fracture involves only the posterior arch of the atlas, it is a distinctly different lesion than the Jefferson fracture of the atlas.

Fracture of the posterior arch of the atlas may occur as an isolated fracture (Fig. 7.3) or in association with other types of cervical spine fractures (Fig. 7.4). Displacement of the fragments may be minimal and oblique views may be necessary to identify the fracture.

The posterior atlantal arch fracture carries no neurologic implications and is stable.

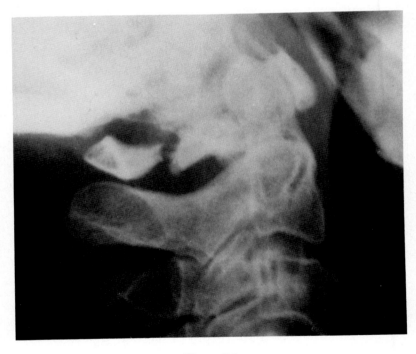

Figure 7.3
Isolated fracture of the posterior arch of the atlas. (Reprinted by permission from Harris, J. H. Jr.: Acute injuries of the spine. *Semin. Roentgenol.* 13:53, 1978.)

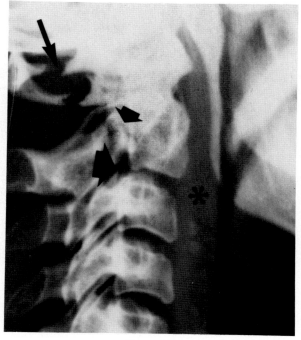

Figure 7.4
Fracture of the posterior arch of the atlas (stemmed arrow) associated with a hangman's fracture of the axis (arrowheads). The asterisk (*) indicates the prevertebral hematoma. (Reprinted by permission from Harris, J. H. Jr. & Harris, W. H.: *The Radiology of Emergency Medicine.* Williams & Wilkins, Baltimore, Md., © 1975.)

C. EXTENSION TEAR-DROP FRACTURE

The fracture involving the anterior inferior corner of the axis, resulting in a separate triangle-shaped fragment pulled off at the insertion of the anterior longitudinal ligament during hyperflexion, has been depicted as the extension tear-drop fracture by Holdsworth (19, 25).

This fracture is characterized radiographically by the typical shape of the separate fragment, the essentially normal alignment of the vertebral bodies, and the common association of pre-existent degenerative arthritis of the cervical spine (Fig. 7.5).

This fracture is pathognomonic of a hyperextension injury. It is stable in flexion because the posterior ligament complex and the interfacetal joints are intact. It is unstable in extension because the anterior longitudinal ligament is separated from the body of the axis by virtue of its

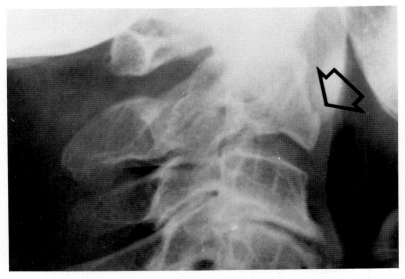

Figure 7.5
Extension tear-drop fracture of the axis (arrow).

attachment on the separate fragment and because of partial separation of the disk from the inferior end-plate of the axis.

D. Hangman's Fracture

Bilateral fracture of the pedicles of the axis, usually associated with dislocation of C_2 on C_3, has been designated "hangman's" fracture by Schneider *et al.* (7) and "traumatic spondylolisthesis" by Garber (57). The close similarity of the pathologic skeletal characteristics of this injury to that caused by judicial hanging has prompted the term "hangman's fracture."

Traumatic spondylolisthesis of the axis is an uncommon lesion. It is usually the result of an automobile accident in which there is abrupt deceleration from a rapid rate of speed. The anatomic basis of the injury relates to the unique structure of the cervico-cranium, which has been described previously, and the inherent weakness in the cervical spine which exists at the C_2–C_3 level, the level of transition between the cervico-cranium and the remainder of the cervical spine.

Head and face injuries are frequently associated with traumatic spondylolisthesis.

The mechanism of injury is predicated upon the cervico-cranium functioning as a unit. The injury occurs as the result of the cervico-cranium being thrown, or forced, into hyperextension at the instant of abrupt deceleration resulting in bilateral fracture of the pedicles of the axis. Because anterior dislocation of the axis on C₃ is invariably present, and because of the frequently associated wedge fracture of C₃, a final rebound flexion component of the mechanism of injury is postulated as well (7, 23, 33, 58).

In the lateral radiograph of the cervical spine, the forward position of the body of the axis is misleading in that it suggests a flexion injury. However, the roentgen characteristics of the injury coupled with an understanding of the mechanism of injury should dispel any notion that traumatic spondylolisthesis is primarily a flexion injury.

Anterior displacement of the body of the axis may be marked (Fig. 7.6) or slight (Fig. 7.4) and the pedicular fracture may be obvious or

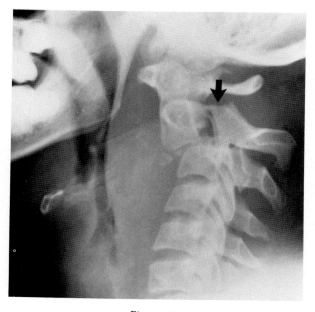

Figure 7.6

Hangman's fracture-dislocation. The bilateral pedicle fracture is indicated by the arrow. The body of the axis and the remainder of the cervico-cranium are dislocated anteriorly. The posterior fragment is dislocated anteriorly so that the inferior articulating facets and articular masses of the axis lie superior to the superior end-plate of C₃. The marked prevertebral soft tissue swelling secondary to the massive hematoma severely compromises the hypopharyngeal airway.

very subtle. The posterior fragment usually retains its normal relationship to the posterior arch of the atlas and C$_3$.

This injury is always accompanied by prevertebral hemorrhage and edema which may compromise the hypopharyngeal airway (Fig. 7.4 and 7.6).

Because of the bilateral pedicle fractures, the hangman's fracture is unstable.

Neurologic complications of traumatic spondylolisthesis are usually not of major consequence. In 14 cases of fracture-dislocation of the axis reported by Cornish (58), only one had quadraparesis. Other neurologic symptoms were diffuse upper limb pain and paresthesia and pain referred to the occipital area. The paucity of neurologic complications is related to the fact that the anteroposterior diameter of the cervical spinal canal is greatest at the axis and that "auto-decompression" of the spinal canal has occurred with the bilateral pedicle fractures.

CHAPTER 8

INJURIES OF THE CERVICO-CRANIUM

As previously noted, the cervico-cranium consists of the occiput, the occipito-atlantal joint, the atlas, the axis, and the atlanto-axial articulation. For practical reasons stemming from the unique anatomic relationships, the distinctive physiologic motions, and the responses to injury that are peculiar to this segment of the central axis, the cervico-cranium has traditionally been considered as a separate entity in the discussion of cervical trauma.

Although the anatomy of the atlas and the axis and the atlanto-axial relationship have been previously described, a few of the anatomic and physiologic characteristics of the atlanto-axial articulation are sufficiently important to an understanding of the roentgen appearance of this area to warrant repetition.

The dens is symmetrically situated between the lateral masses of the atlas and serves as the pivotal point for rotation of the atlas on the axis. The corresponding articular facets of the atlas and the axis (the lateral atlanto-axial joints) are each convex. The medial and lateral margins of these articular surfaces are very closely symmetrical, *i.e.,* the lateral margin of the lateral articular facet of C_1 is superimposed upon that of C_2 (Fig. 8.1).

Fielding (9) has shown, cineradiographically, that during rotation of the head, the skull and atlas turn as a unit with the atlas pivoting on the axis, about the dens. Simply stated, C_1 rotates on C_2. During rotation, the following physiologic changes in the relationship of the lateral

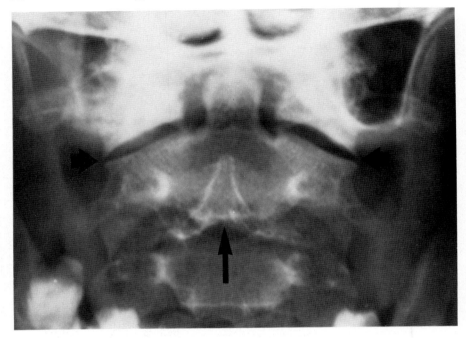

Figure 8.1
Open-mouth projection of the normal atlanto-axial articulation. The lateral margins of the contiguous articulating facets of the atlas and axis are precisely superimposed (broad arrows). The bifid spinous process of the axis is a midline structure (stemmed arrow).

masses of the atlas and axis occur. (*a*) As the head rotates in one direction, the contralateral lateral mass of the atlas rotates forward and medially and becomes rectangular in appearance. The distance between this lateral mass and the dens decreases and the medial and lateral margins of the inferior facet of the atlas lie medial to their counterparts of the axis (Fig. 8.2). (*b*) The lateral mass of the atlas on the side of the direction of the rotation moves posteriorly and becomes truncated in configuration. The distance between this lateral mass of the atlas and the dens remains unaltered or decreases slightly and the margins of the articular facets become asymmetrical (Fig. 8.2).

As rotation increases toward maximum, the convex inferior articulating facets of the atlas glide forward and backward on the convex superior facets of the axis. Whereas in neutral position, these facets are in apposition at the highest point of their convex surfaces and an open joint space is clearly evident (Fig. 8.1), with rotation the high point of the inferior facet of the atlas drops below the high point of the superior facet of the axis and the lateral atlanto-axial joint spaces become narrow or obliterated in direct proportion to the amount of rotation. When the atlas rotates off the high point of the convex articulating surfaces of the axis, the total vertical height of the atlanto-axial complex decreases (Fig. 8.3). This has been called "vertical approximation" or "telescoping" by Fielding (9) and is one of the physiologic motions at this level.

Another physiologic effect, which occurs with increasing rotation, relates to the axis. During the first half of the rotational range, the axis remains stationary. With further rotation of the head, the axis rotates in

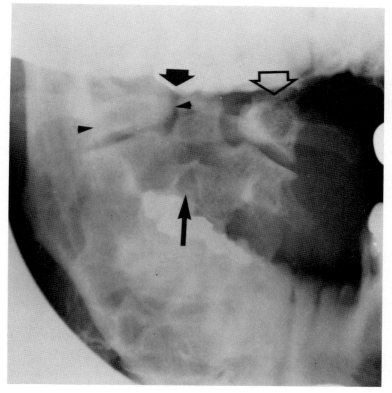

Figure 8.2
Open-mouth projection of the normal atlanto-axial articulation during moderate rotation to the left. The right lateral mass of the atlas has rotated anteriorly and appears to have increased in transverse diameter (small arrowheads). The distance between this lateral mass and the dens is narrowed (solid arrow) and the margins of its articulating facet lie medial to those of the superior facet of the axis. The left lateral mass of the atlas (open arrow) has rotated posteriorly and is truncated in configuration. The margins of the left lateral atlanto-axial joint are asymmetrical. The spinous process of the axis (stemmed arrow) remains in the midline.

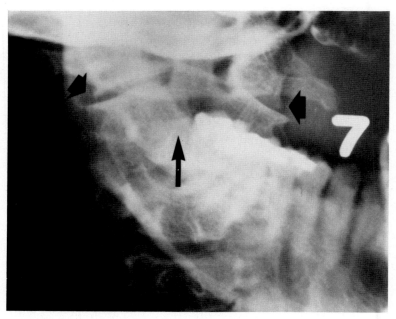

Figure 8.3
Normal atlanto-axial articulation in marked rotation. Narrowing and obliteration of the lateral joint spaces due to vertical approximation are indicated by the solid arrows. The asymmetry of the margins of these joints is physiologic. The spinous process of the axis (stemmed arrow) is deviated to the right of the midline indicating rotation of the axis in the same direction as the rotation of the head.

the same direction and its bifid spinous process deviates away from the midline in the opposite direction (Fig. 8.3).

Lateral tilt or bending is simply allowing the head to deviate off the midline to one side or the other. For the purposes of definition and demonstration, lateral tilt will be assumed to be a pure motion completely devoid of any rotational component. (Pure lateral tilt is difficult to accomplish and probably occurs naturally only rarely.)

During lateral tilt, the skull and atlas move as a unit and glide from the midline toward the side of the tilt. For example, if the head is tilted to the left, the atlas glides to the left with respect to the axis. Consequently, the space between the right lateral mass and the dens decreases and the space between the dens and the left lateral mass of the axis increases slightly. The margins of the contiguous articular facets of the atlas and axis become asymmetrical (Fig. 8.4).

The axis (C_2) and the subjacent vertebrae rotate during lateral tilt. This normal, physiologic component of lateral bending (tilt) occurs early during lateral bending and the rotation is in the direction of the tilt. For example, if the head is tilted to the left, the axis rotates to the left causing the bifid spinous process of the axis to deviate to the right of the midline. It may be surprising to learn that the axis rotates during lateral bending and that it occurs earlier in lateral bending than during rotation. However, this fact has been conclusively demonstrated by Fielding (9) and is illustrated in Figure 8.5. The importance of this physiologic fact will become evident in the discussion of atlanto-axial injury.

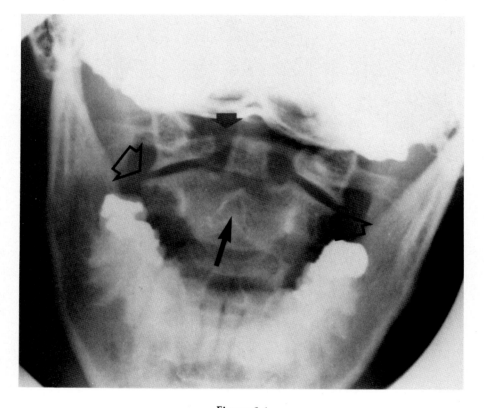

Figure 8.4
Normal atlanto-axial articulation in minimal lateral tilt to the left. The atlas has glided to the left. The space between the right lateral mass of the atlas and the dens has decreased (solid arrow) while that on the left has widened. The lateral margins of the lateral atlanto-axial joint spaces are physiologically asymmetrical (open arrows). At this minimal degree of tilt, the axis has not rotated and its spinous process (stemmed arrows) remains in the midline.

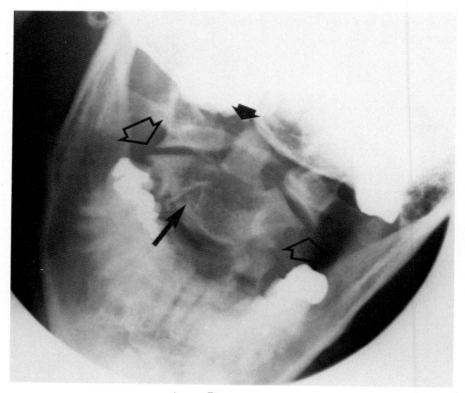

Figure 8.5
Normal atlanto-axial articulation in moderate lateral tilt to the left. The physiologic changes illustrated in Figure 8.4 are accentuated. In addition, with greater tilt, physiologic rotation of the axis to the left has resulted in its spinous process (stemmed arrow) being deviated to the right of the midline.

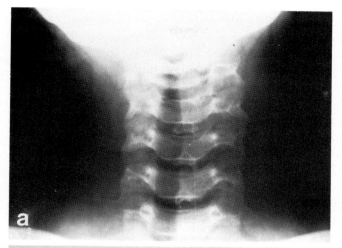

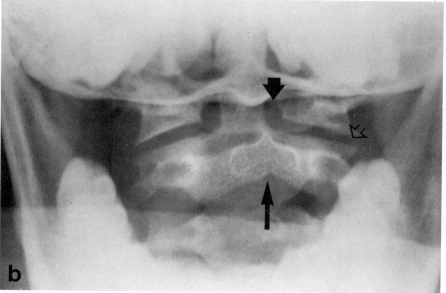

Figure 8.6

Torticollis with the head rotated and tilted to the *right* (a). In the open-mouth projection (b), the atlas is shifted and rotated to the right causing a decrease in width of the space between the dens and the left lateral mass of C_1 (short arrow), an increase in the width of the left lateral mass, and asymmetry of the lateral margin of the lateral atlanto-axial joint (open arrow). The right lateral mass of the axis appears truncated in configuration by being posteriorly rotated. Rotation of the axis to the right is indicated by displacement of its bifid spinous process to the left of the midline (stemmed arrow).

The preceding review of the physiologic motions that occur in the cervico-cranium during rotation and lateral bending of the head is essential to a proper evaluation of the frequently perplexing radiographic appearance of the atlanto-axial articulation. It is unfortunate that such terms as "unilateral offset" and "bilateral offset" (59, 60) have been used to describe atlanto-axial relationships which are physiologic because through common usage, these terms are accepted by many as indicating a pathologic state. "Subluxation" and "dislocation" are, by definition, abnormal terms, but the radiographic relationships of C_1–C_2 to which they have been ascribed are more often normal than abnormal. "Offset" has, also by common usage, come to be synonymous with abnormality. It has been established that unilateral and bilateral offset *alone* are not pathologic and should not be considered signs of subluxation or dislocation at the atlanto-axial articulation (10, 33, 61, 62). Displacement of one or both lateral masses of the atlas in conjunction with atlantal fractures has been discussed previously.

It is hoped that by describing the physiologic motions at the atlanto-axial articulation and by illustrating the roentgen appearance of these motions, the terms "offset," "rotational subluxation" and "physiologic dislocation" have been shown to be not only imprecise, but frankly misleading.

Fielding and Hawkins (33) have used the term "rotational displacement" to describe the physiologic changes at the atlanto-axial articulation. This term describes more accurately the events that occur during rotation and lateral bending, and conveys no implication of abnormality, thus leaving the significance of the roentgen findings to interpretation in light of the clinical situation. Therefore, unless there are definite roentgen signs of skeletal or soft tissue injury in the cervico-cranium, the significance of alterations in alignment of the atlas and the axis, *i.e.,* "rotational displacement," must depend upon the clinical findings.

A. TORTICOLLIS ("WRY-NECK")

Torticollis is a clinical condition, frequently seen in childhood and early adolescence, which may occur spontaneously, follow minor trauma to the head or neck, or be associated with acute infection of the face or neck. It is characterized, clinically, by tilting of the head in one direction and simultaneous rotation of the head in the opposite direction, and is characterized radiographically by atlanto-axial rotary displacement.

The etiology of the deformity is unknown. The pathophysiology, which is described as "locking" or "catching" (63) of the interfacetal joints at some point during rotation of the atlas on the axis, is usually self-limited, and the deformity usually reverses spontaneously. Occasionally, however, the deformity may persist, in which event the altered relationship of C_1 and C_2 is referred to as atlanto-axial rotary *fixation* (33).

The roentgen evaluation of the patient with torticollis is challenging because the painful deformity makes positioning of the patient difficult and, consequently, interpretation of the roentgenograms frequently perplexing.

No attempt to straighten the head and neck in order to obtain a "good," *i.e.,* straight, antero-posterior radiograph should be attempted. To do so aggravates the patient's pain and also diminishes, or eliminates, the characteristic roentgen signs of torticollis.

The lateral tilt and rotation of the head that occur in torticollis result in physiologic movements of the atlas and the axis which have been described and illustrated earlier in this chapter (Figs. 8.2–8.5). In torticollis, however, these movements are the result of the underlying etiology of the torticollis, be it congenital or acquired. The lateral tilt of the head causes the atlas to shift, or glide, laterally with respect to the dens in the same direction as the tilt of the head, and causes the axis to rotate in the same direction also. The associated rotation of the head causes the atlas to rotate also and in the same direction.

The roentgen signs of torticollis, then, are the sum of the effects of lateral tilt and rotation of the head upon the atlas and axis. For these reasons, therefore, Fielding's term "atlanto-axial rotary displacement" (33) seems to be the most appropriate designation for the roentgen findings because it contains no connotation of a pathologic condition and leaves the diagnosis of torticollis to be based upon the clinical picture.

The roentgen findings include asymmetry of the spaces between the dens and the articular masses of the axis, asymmetry of the lateral margins of the lateral atlanto-axial joints, increase in transverse diameter (width) of the anteriorly rotated articular mass of the atlas, and displacement of the bifid spinous process of the axis from the midline in the direction opposite that of the torticollis deformity (Figs. 8.6 and 8.7).

In the lateral radiograph, the rotation and lateral tilt of the atlas and axis in torticollis result in a loss of definition of the normal atlanto-axial anatomy (Fig. 8.8).

Fractures and dislocations of the cervico-cranium are not commonly encountered clinically because of the associated high mortality rate. Nearly 81% of fatal cervical spine injuries reported by Alker *et al.* (64) involve the cervico-cranium. Davis *et al.* (65), analyzing the pathologic findings in a series of 50 fatal cases of cranio-spinal injury, indicate that there is a high incidence of cord damage with these injuries, and that

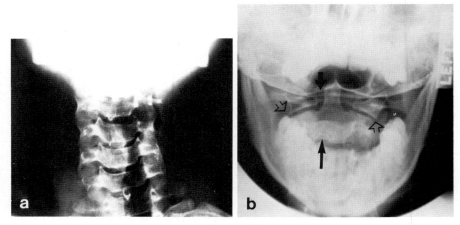

Figure 8.7

Torticollis with the head rotated and tilted to the *left* (a). In the open-mouth projection (b), the atlas has shifted and rotated to the left resulting in a decrease in the width of the space between its right lateral mass and the dens (short arrow), an apparent increase in the transverse diameter of the right lateral mass because of its anterior rotation, and asymmetry of the lateral margins of the lateral atlanto-axial joints (open arrows). The left lateral mass of the axis appears truncated because of its posterior rotation. Rotation of the axis to the left is indicated by displacement of its spinous process to the right of the midline (stemmed arrow).

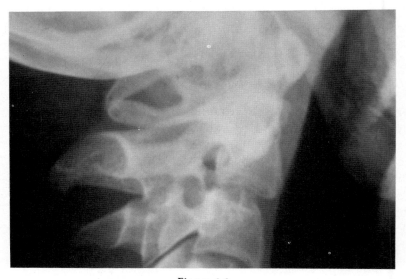

Figure 8.8

Torticollis. Rotation and lateral tilt of the atlas and axis result in loss of definition of the normal anatomy of the cervico-cranium in lateral projection.

cervico-cranial fractures or dislocations are much more frequently encountered in fatal accidents than are fractures of the lower cervical segments.

Retropharyngeal hematoma, frequently sufficient to occlude the airway, is invariably associated with fractures or dislocations at the atlanto-occipital or the atlanto-axial level (33, 64, 65).

It is a commonly held misconception that acute traumatic disruption of the transverse atlantal ligament is a frequent cause of atlanto-axial instability or dislocation. Acute rupture of the transverse ligament is rare (11, 65) and may be presumed if, following severe trauma, the ADI exceeds 3 mm in adults. If the ADI exceeds 5 mm it may be assumed that both the transverse atlantal and the alar ligaments are ruptured.

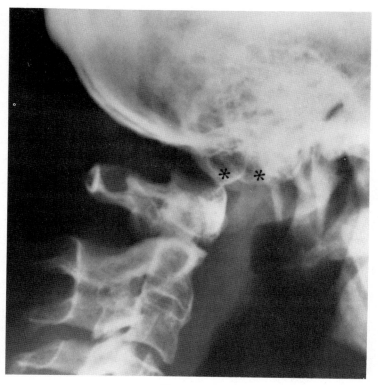

Figure 8.9
Fatal anterior occipito-atlantal dislocation with associated atlanto-axial rotary dislocation. The occipital condyles (*) are anteriorly dislocated with respect to the superior facets of the atlas. The atlas has rotated about the dens and the anterior arch of the atlas is obscured by its anteriorly rotated right lateral mass. The posterior arch and the spinous process of the atlas are foreshortened due to the rotation.

More common causes for atlanto-axial instability include anomalies and fractures of the dens and rheumatoid arthritis (33).

B. DISLOCATION

Dislocation at the atlanto-occipital level, and atlanto-axial rotary dislocation, where the atlas is rotated approximately 90° on the axis, are rarely seen clinically, because they are incompatible with life (Fig. 8.9).

C. FRACTURE

Compression fracture of the atlas (Jefferson fracture), the isolated fracture of the posterior arch of C_1, and the hangman's fracture have all been described elsewhere.

Fractures of the dens have been classified by Anderson and D'Alonzo (66) on the basis of the location of the fracture (Fig. 8.10). Type I, which is an oblique avulsion fracture of the tip of the dens at the site of attachment of the alar ligament, is an uncommon injury. This fracture is stable and is not complicated by nonunion.

The Type II fracture occurs at the junction of the dens and the body of the axis. It is the most common of the dens fractures, and is frequently complicated by failure of union. Schatzker *et al.* (67), in analyzing 37

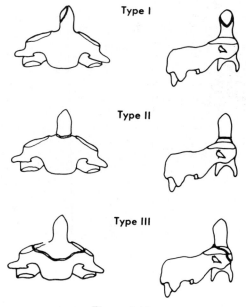

Figure 8.10
Classification of dens fractures according to Anderson and D'Alonzo (66).

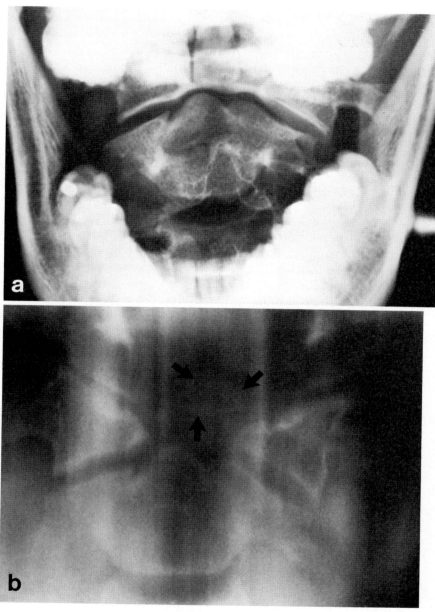

Figure 8.11
Os odontoideum. In the plain open-mouth projection (a), the separate ossicle is obscured by the superimposed incisor teeth and anterior arch of the atlas. The appearance of the superior aspect of the body of the axis suggests the presence of an os odontoideum. The separate ossicle (arrows) is visible in the frontal tomogram (b).

cases of fracture of the dens, reported an incidence of 64% nonunion over-all, and in those fractures with posterior displacement or more than 5 mm displacement, approximately 100% nonunion.

Fractures of the Type II variety are initially unstable and should be treated with skull traction as an emergency procedure to avoid the danger of cord compression (67).

The Type III fracture extends into the body of the axis, is stable, and characteristically heals.

The roentgen diagnosis of the fracture of the dens is frequently difficult. Failure of fusion of the dens and the body of the axis (Fig. 8.11) and the os odontoideum, a congenital or acquired (68) condition in which the tip of the dens is separated from the body of the axis by a wide gap, may simulate a fracture. The Mach effect at the junction of the base of the dens and the body of the axis, caused by superimposition of the anterior arch of the atlas (Fig. 8.12), frequently resembles a fracture line. The Mach effect changes with alterations of positioning and is not associated with prevertebral soft tissue swelling.

The fracture line of non- or minimally displaced Type II (Fig. 8.13) or Type III fractures is commonly difficult to identify and tomograms made in frontal and lateral projections are invariably required to establish the diagnosis. The most conspicuous sign of a dens fracture on the

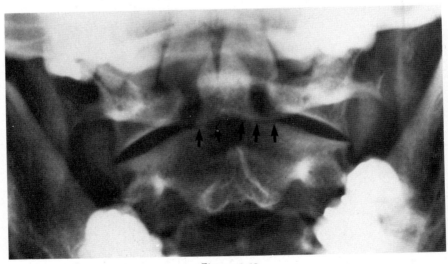

Figure 8.12
The superimposition of the inferior margin of the anterior arch of the atlas upon the base of the dens results in a radiolucent Mach effect which closely simulates a fracture line (arrows).

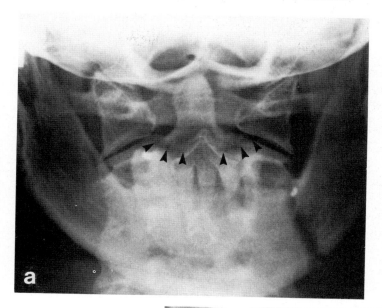

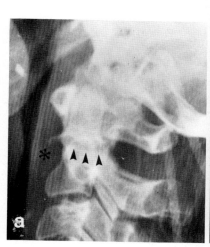
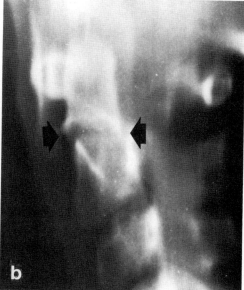

Figure 8.13

Type II fracture of the dens in a patient with multiple injuries, including a mandibular fracture (arrow). The dens fracture line (arrowheads) is very subtle in both the open-mouth (a) and lateral (b) projections. In the lateral radiograph a thin bony fragment, which arises from the dens, projects into the prevertebral soft tissues which are abnormally thickened (*) by the associated hematoma. The fracture line (arrows) and displacement of the fragments are obvious in the lateral tomogram (c).

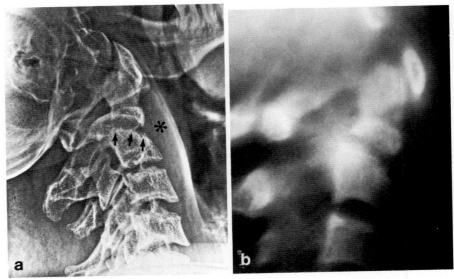

Figure 8.14
This Type III dens fracture was poorly visualized on plain frontal and lateral radiographs. The fracture line, which extends into the body of the axis (small arrows) and the prevertebral soft tissue swelling (*) are clearly evident in the xerograph (a). The displaced fracture is obvious in the lateral tomogram (b). (Courtesy of William E. Jobe, M.D., Swedish Medical Center, Denver, Colorado.)

plain lateral radiograph is frequently the prevertebral soft tissue swelling anterior to the atlanto-axial level caused by the hematoma associated with the fracture.

Flexion and extension views of the cervical spine are contraindicated when a dens fracture is suspected in order to avoid potentially fatal displacement.

Xeroradiography is valuable in the demonstration of fractures of the dens (Fig. 8.14).

References

1. Von Torklus, D. & Gehle, W.: *The Upper Cervical Spine.* Grune & Stratton, New York, 1972.
2. Brocker, J. E. W.: Die Occipital-Cervical-Gegend. Thieme, Stuttgart, 1955. As cited by Von Torklus & Gehle, Reference 1.
3. Locke, G. R., Gardner, J. E. & Van Epps, E. F.: Atlas-dens interval (ADI) in children. *Am. J. Roentgenol. Radium Ther. Nucl. Med.* 97:135, 1966.
4. Cattell, H. S. & Filtzer, D. L.: Pseudosubluxation and other normal variations of the cervical spine in children. *J. Bone Joint Surg.* 47-A:1295, 1965.
5. Caffey, J.: *Pediatric X-ray Diagnosis,* 6th Ed. Yearbook Medical Publishers, Chicago, 1972.
6. Swischuk, L. E.: Anterior dislocation of C_2 in children: physiologic or pathologic? *Radiology* 122:759, 1977.
7. Schneider, R. C., Livingston, K. E., Cave, A. J. E. & Hamilton, G.: "Hangman's fracture" of the cervical spine. *J. Neurosurg.* 22:141, 1965.
8. Coutts, M. B.: Atlanto-epistropheal subluxations. *Arch. Surg.* 29:297, 1934.
9. Fielding, J. W.: Cineroentgenography of the normal cervical spine. *J. Bone Joint Surg.* 39-A:1280, 1957.
10. Hohl, M.: Normal motions in the upper portion of the cervical spine. *J. Bone Joint Surg.* 46-A:1777, 1964.
11. Fielding, J. W., Cochran, G. V. B., Lawsing, J. F. III & Hohl, M.: Tears of the transverse ligament of the atlas. *J. Bone Joint Surg.* 56-A:1683, 1974.
12. Hinck, V. C. & Hopkins, C. E.: Measurement of the atlanto-dental interval in the adult. *Radiology* 84:945, 1964.
13. Hay, P. D.: Measurement of the soft tissues of the neck. In Lusted, L. B. & Keats, T. E. (Eds.): *Atlas of Roentgenographic Measurement,* 3rd Ed. Yearbook Medical Publishers, Chicago, 1972.
14. Fielding, J. W.: Normal and selected abnormal motions of the cervical spine from the second cervical vertebra to the seventh cervical vertebra based on cineroentgenography. *J. Bone Joint Surg.* 46-A:1779, 1964.
15. Weir, D. C.: Roentgenographic signs of cervical injury. *Clin. Orthopaed.* 109:9, 1975.
16. Edeiken, J.: Personal communication.
17. Abel, M. S.: *Occult Traumatic Lesions of the Cervical Vertebrae.* Warren H. Green, St. Louis, 1971.
18. Vines, F. S.: The significance of "occult" fractures of the cervical spine. *Am. J. Roentgenol. Radium Ther. Nucl. Med.* 107:493, 1969.
19. Holdsworth, F.: Fractures, dislocations and fracture-dislocations of the spine. *J. Bone Joint Surg.* 52-A:1534, 1970.
20. Beatson, T. R.: Fractures and dislocations of the cervical spine. *J. Bone Joint Surg.* 45-B:21, 1963.
21. Whitley, J. E. & Forsyth, H. F.: The classification of cervical spine injuries. *Am. J. Roentgenol. Radium Ther. Nucl. Med.* 83:633, 1960.
22. Apley, A. G.: Fractures of the spine. *Ann. R. Coll. Surg. Engl.* 46:210, 1970.
23. Babcock, J. L.: Cervical spine injuries. *Arch. Surg.* 111:646, 1976.
24. Cheshire, D. J. E.: The stability of the cervical spine following the conservative treatment of fractures and fracture-dislocations. *Paraplegia* 7:193, 1969.
25. Holdsworth, F. W.: Early orthopaedic treatment of patients with spinal injuries. In Harris, P. (Ed.): *Spinal Injuries.* Morrison & Gibb, London, 1963.
26. Bedbrook, G. M.: Stability of spinal fractures and fracture-dislocations. *Paraplegia* 9:23, 1971.
27. Rothman, R. H. & Simeone, F. A.: *The Spine.* W. B. Saunders, Philadelphia, 1975.

28. Petrie, J. G.: Flexion injuries of the cervical spine. *J. Bone Joint Surg.* 46-A:1800, 1964.

29. Roaf, R.: A study of the mechanics of spinal injuries. *J. Bone Joint Surg.* 42-B:810, 1960.

30. Garber, W. N., Fisher, R. G. & Holfman, H. W.: Vertebrectomy and fusion for "tear-drop fracture" of the cervical spine. *J. Trauma* 9:887, 1969.

31. Schneider, R. C. & Kahn, E. A.: Chronic neurologic sequelae of acute trauma to the spine and spinal cord. Part I. The significance of the acute-flexion or "tear-drop" fracture-dislocation of the cervical spine. *J. Bone Joint Surg.* 38-A:985, 1956.

32. Feuer, H.: Management of acute spine and spinal cord injuries. *Arch. Surg.* 111:638, 1976.

33. Fielding, J. W. & Hawkins, R. J.: Roentgenographic diagnosis of the injured neck. In *A.A.O.S. Instructional Course Lectures,* Vol. XXV; Chapter 7, pages 149–170. C. V. Mosby, St. Louis, 1976.

34. Selecki, B. R. & Williams, H. B. L.: *Injuries to the Cervical Spine and Cord in Man.* Australasian Medical Publishing Co., New South Wales, 1970.

35. Taylor, R. G. & Gleave, J. R. W.: Injuries to the cervical spine. *Proc. R. Soc. Med.* 55:1053, 1962.

36. Cramer, F. & McGowan, F. J.: The role of the nucleus pulposus in the pathogenesis of the so-called "recoil" injuries of the spinal cord. *Surg. Gynecol. Obstet.* 79:516, 1944.

37. Rogers, W. A.: Fractures and dislocations of the cervical spine. *J. Bone Joint Surg.* 39-A:341, 1957.

38. Jackson, R.: Up-dating the neck. *Trauma* 1:9, 1970.

39. Stringa, G.: Traumatic lesions of the cervical spine—statistics, mechanism, classification. In *Proceedings of the IXth Congress of the International Society of Orthopaedic Surgery & Traumatology.* Imprimerie des Sciences, Brussels, 1963.

40. Braakman, R. & Penning, L.: The hyperflexion sprain of the cervical spine. *Radiol. Clin. Biol.* 37:309, 1968.

41. King, D. M.: Fractures and dislocations of the cervical part of the spine. *Austr. N. Z. J. Surg.* 37:57, 1967.

42. Gosch, H. H., Gooding, E. & Schneider, R. C.: An experimental study of cervical spine and cord injuries. *J. Trauma* 12:570, 1972.

43. Schneider, R. C.: A syndrome in acute cervical spine injuries for which early operation is indicated. *J. Neurosurg.* 8:360, 1951.

44. Schneider, R. C.: The syndrome of acute anterior spinal cord injury. *J. Neurosurg.* 12:95, 1955.

45. Schneider, R. C.: Cervical spine and spinal cord injuries. *Mich. Med.* 773–786, November 1964.

46. Braakman, R. & Vinken, P. J.: Unilateral facet interlocking in the lower cervical spine. *J. Bone Joint Surg.* 49-B:249, 1967.

47. Smith, G. R., Beckly, D. E. & Abel, M. S.: Articular mass fracture: a neglected cause of post-traumatic pain? *Clin. Radiol.* 27:335, 1976.

48. Jefferson, G.: Fracture of the atlas vertebra. Report of four cases, and a review of those previously recorded. *Br. J. Surg.* 7:407, 1920.

49. Marar, B. C.: The pattern of neurologic damage as an aid to the diagnosis of the mechanism in cervical spine injuries. *J. Bone Joint Surg.* 56-A:1648, 1974.

50. Taylor, A. R. & Blackwood, W.: Paraplegia in hyperextension cervical injuries with normal radiographic appearances. *J. Bone Joint Surg.* 30-B:245, 1948.

51. Taylor, A. R.: The mechanism of injury to the spinal cord in the neck without damage to the vertebral column. *J. Bone Joint Surg.* 33-B:543, 1951.

52. Schneider, R. C. & Pantek, H.: The syndrome of acute central cervical cord injury with special reference to the mechanisms involved in hyperextension injuries of the cervical spine. *J. Neurosurg.* 11:546, 1954.

53. Schneider, R. C., Thompson, J. M. & Bebin, J.: The syndrome of acute central cervical spinal cord injury. *J. Neurol. Neurosurg. Psychiatry* 21:216, 1958.

54. Schneider, R. C.: Chronic neurologic sequelae of acute trauma to the spine and spinal cord. Part V. The syndrome of acute central cervical spine injury followed by chronic anterior cervical cord injury (or compression) syndrome. *J. Bone Joint Surg.* 42-A:253, 1960.

55. Forsyth, H. F.: Extension injuries of the cervical spine. *J. Bone Joint Surg.* 46-A:1792, 1964.

56. Sinbert, S. E. & Berman, M. S.: Fracture of the posterior arch of the atlas. *J. A. M. A.* 114:1996, 1940.

57. Garber, J. N.: Abnormalities of the atlas and axis vertebrae—congenital and traumatic. *J. Bone Joint Surg.* 46-A:1792, 1964.

58. Cornish, B. L.: Traumatic spondylolisthesis of the axis. *J. Bone Joint Surg.* 50-B:31, 1968.

59. Jacobson, G. & Alder, D. C.: An evaluation of lateral atlanto-axial displacement in injuries of the cervical spine. *Radiology* 61:355, 1961.

60. Jacobson, G. & Alder, D. C.: Examination of the atlanto-axial joint following injury with particular emphasis on rotational subluxation. *Am. J. Roentgenol. Radium Ther. Nucl. Med.* 76:1081, 1956.

61. Paul, L. W. & Moir, W. W.: Non-pathologic variations in relationship of the upper cervical vertebrae. *Radiology* 62:519, 1949.

62. Hohl, M. & Baker, H. R.: The atlanto-axial joint. *J. Bone Joint Surg.* 46-A:1739, 1964.

63. Schmorl, G. & Junghanns, H.: *The Human Spine in Health and Disease,* 2nd Am. Ed. Grune & Stratton, New York, 1971.

64. Alker, G. J., Oh, Y. S., Leslie, E. V., Lehotay, J., Panaro, V. A. & Eschner, E. G.: Postmortem radiology of head and neck injuries in fatal traffic accidents. *Radiology* 114:611, 1975.

65. Davis, D., Bohlman, H., Walker, A. E., Fisher, R. & Robinson, R.: The pathological findings in fatal cranio-spinal injuries. *J. Neurosurg.* 34:603, 1971.

66. Anderson, L. D. & D'Alonzo, R. T.: Fractures of the odontoid process of the axis. *J. Bone Joint Surg.* 56-A:1663, 1974.

67. Schatzker, J., Rorabeck, C. H. & Waddell, J. P.: Fractures of the dens (odontoid process); an analysis of 37 cases. *J. Bone Joint Surg.* 53-B: 392, 1971.

68. Fielding, J. W. & Griffin, P. P.: Os odontoideum: an acquired lesion. *J. Bone Joint Surg.* 56-A:187, 1974.

INDEX*

* Page numbers in bold type refer to pages
with illustrations.